Get Well
Stay Well

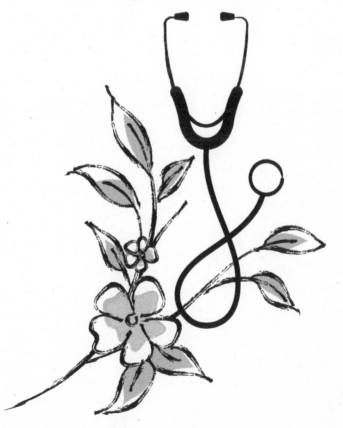

Also by Dr Gemma Newman

The Plant Power Doctor:
A Simple Prescription for a Healthier You

Get Well
Stay Well

The six healing health habits you need to know

Dr Gemma Newman

EBURY
PRESS

Ebury Press, an imprint of Ebury Publishing
20 Vauxhall Bridge Road
London SW1V 2SA

Ebury Press is part of the Penguin Random House group of companies
whose addresses can be found at global.penguinrandomhouse.com

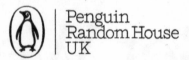

Copyright © Dr Gemma Newman 2023
Illustrations by Rebecca Wheele

Dr Gemma Newman has asserted her right to be identified as the author of
this Work in accordance with the Copyright, Designs and Patents Act 1988

First published by Ebury Press in 2023

www.penguin.co.uk

A CIP catalogue record for this book is available from the British Library

ISBN 9781529107692

Typeset in 11/16pt Baskerville MT Pro by Jouve (UK), Milton Keynes
Printed and bound in Great Britain by Clays Ltd, Elcograf S.p.A.

The authorised representative in the EEA is Penguin Random House
Ireland, Morrison Chambers, 32 Nassau Street, Dublin D02 YH68

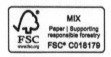

Penguin Random House is committed to a sustainable future
for our business, our readers and our planet. This book is made
from Forest Stewardship Council® certified paper.

This book is dedicated to you. It takes courage to make changes on your journey towards more health and happiness.

In the wise words of Goldie Hawn: 'Giving back is as good for you as it is for those you are helping, because giving gives you purpose. When you have a purpose-driven life, you're a happier person.'

Thank you for giving me a chance to be a part of your journey.

Contents

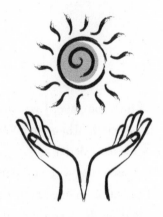

Introduction

The Time for Change Is Now

One day a few years ago, I was driving home from a busy day in clinic when I realised something: most of my patients were not getting better.

In my clinic, I was tinkering with my patient's medications, checking their blood pressure, giving them medications to chip away at their blood sugar levels, prescribing them tablets to ease their pain – *but nobody was actually getting better.*

I thought to myself bleakly, 'Have I actually helped anyone today?' In all my years of clinical practice, I had never felt more powerless.

I realised more of my patients than ever were struggling financially, emotionally and physically. It felt like I was trying to mop up the water on the floor from a bathtub already overflowing with water – a never-ending and impossible task. *What do I need to do?* I thought. *I need to help them pull the plug. Unblock the drain. Let the water drain away.* But *how?*

The truth is that many of our life circumstances are beyond our control: our genes, the colour of our skin, the family we are born into, our childhood experiences, infections we have been exposed to, our schooling, our parents, our friends and mentors and much more. All these things play an important part in our health, and they always have. Medical, mental and social problems are nothing new. But in recent years, I have seen more and more young people struggling to feel well. People that I'd rarely see in my clinic office are now regular patients, presenting with hard-to-define symptoms, a feeling of anxiety, and an absence of the energy they need to get through their days.

Why are more young patients coming to see me, struggling with chronic illnesses? By 'young' I mean teenagers through to patients in their thirties and forties – not the age demographic I expect to see so frequently – weighed down by the illnesses more commonly associated with older demographics. They feel, unsurprisingly, stressed, disconnected and demoralised about their health. When they should be in the prime of life, my patients are struggling.

A report from 2021 on the prevalence of chronic pain in England found that the proportion of people aged 16 to 34 affected by what experts call 'high-impact chronic pain' (pain so severe that it leaves them struggling to work, interact socially and look after themselves) rose dramatically between 2011 and 2017, from 21 per cent to 34 per cent.[1] It is really worrying to me that there is such a large increase in chronic pain in young adults, one that is not seen in any other age group.

People of lower income, women and ethnic minorities feel the impact of chronic pain the most.[1] Fibromyalgia, irritable bowel syndrome, inflammatory bowel disease, chronic fatigue, depression, endometriosis and autoimmune diseases can all contribute. There are other reasons for chronic pain too – like declining levels of physical activity, chronic lack of sleep, reduced feelings of connection and wider socioeconomic trends like job insecurity or an inability to buy a home.

Some of my patients are experiencing social and economic exclusion in a world that does not easily accept people with differences; those who are carrying extra weight, living with ADHD, are autistic or those who have a non-binary gender identity are just a few examples of this.[2,3,4]

Young people are not faring much better across the pond; over half of Americans between 18 and 34 years old are living with a chronic medical condition, according to a recent report from the

Centers for Disease Control and Prevention (CDC).[5] These conditions include obesity, depression, high blood pressure and asthma. The 2020 pandemic was also a wake-up call when it comes to chronic disease. So many people now also live with ill health due to long COVID, which has no clear cure and attacks the body, mind and nervous system. Many patients, young and old, feel forced to look beyond medicine for answers, and so they will try all kinds of unproven and sometimes expensive routes to recovery.

The problems we are facing as a society affect us mentally as well as physically. According to the charity Mind, one in four of us suffers from a mental health problem every year.[6] This means the chances are that we will all be affected by mental health issues, or love someone who suffers from them; that's the simple truth. My father was a good and kind soul but he suffered from severe depression during his lifetime. He experienced attempted suicide, medications, electroconvulsive therapy, hospital admissions and ultimately premature death from heart disease. Smoking and physiological stress, which he was prone to because of his depression, were big factors at play when understanding the role heart disease had in his untimely death.

Every day when I am working in my practice, I see the impact of mental health on the body. As a GP, I would say that stress and mental health factor in at least 80 per cent of the patients that I see.

The Mental Health Foundation tells us that one in ten children suffers from mental health problems, including depression, anxiety and conduct disorders.[7] Rates of self-harm are also on the rise. The Adult Psychiatric Morbidity Survey (APMS) provides England's national statistics – it tells us that one in six adults has a common mental disorder (CMD): one in five women, and one in eight men. This includes depression, generalised anxiety disorder (GAD), panic disorder, phobias, social anxiety disorder, obsessive-compulsive disorder (OCD) and post-traumatic stress disorder (PTSD).[8]

The reasons for mental health problems are complex, and for many people it involves a combination of factors including childhood trauma, a lack of coping strategies, reactions to individual traumatic events, social isolation, severe or long-term stress, long-term health conditions, and other genetic or environmental factors. When you are experiencing a mental illness, it is important to seek professional help. Your GP should be able to direct you to talking therapies and will also be able to prescribe medications that could be an important therapeutic tool in managing your condition. There is no shame in taking medication for mental health struggles, just as there is no shame in taking a tablet to help control blood pressure.

Do any of these issues resonate with you? Have you noticed the impact of some of these problems in your own life?

Modern medicine is truly on the back foot. It is not easy to understand why mental health problems, but also physical conditions such as endometriosis and inflammatory bowel diseases – even bowel cancers – seem to be rising in the younger generation.[9-11]

The questions I had on my journey that night continued to swirl in my mind. Why are my patients not getting better? I had to find out. How could I help if I didn't know why?

I started looking for trends in large populations of people. Perhaps what I was seeing in clinic was relevant on a bigger scale? It turns out the rise in chronic health conditions I was seeing in my patients is mirrored in communities across the Western world.[12] Some researchers have attributed the rise in autoimmune diseases in younger people to increasing consumption of fast food.[13] This is one of the reasons why focusing on healthy wholefoods is vital. But it is not the only reason.

Our genetics have not changed significantly in the last 30

years, and therefore other factors are clearly also at work. Over the 20 years I have treated patients, I have come to see clearly that:

- ❈ What we eat impacts our health.
- ❈ How we live impacts our health.
- ❈ What we experience in our lives and how we process it impacts our health.

Why an open-minded approach to healthcare is essential

Over the decades, I've been on a mission to prevent illness at its root cause, wherever possible. It became clear to me that my medical degree had some limitations despite my years of training. I have spent years studying not only medicine, but also nutrition, psychotherapy and holistic approaches, determined to tackle the common chronic health issues my patients struggle with. Sometimes these approaches have garnered criticism, either from people who say it is impossible to change social determinants of our health, or from those who say complementary therapies are useless. I remain open-minded. I feel it is helpful to share some of the studies – done over the years by researchers in the fields of nutrition, psychology and medicine – that have helped guide my advice in this book. The reason for this is simple. Being able to interpret the research that is published in peer-reviewed journals helps us to minimise the influence of bias. Even the best-intentioned scientists can't escape personal bias. If we found something that worked for us, it is far more likely we would seek out information that confirms our world view. This is true for all humans.

In the scientific community, researchers must show an

awareness of bias, attempt an objective study, and allow review of their research by other scientists in their field before printing their research. This is an important process which helps to make the information we learn from studies more trustworthy. When results are duplicated by independent research teams, our conclusions about whether something works or not are strengthened. This process is not foolproof. But the scientific method does help to provide a standardised approach to conducting experiments and, in so doing, not only improves their results, but also our confidence in their conclusions.

I believe it is also important to recognise 20 years of clinical experience, and the intuition that results from that hyper-specific type of pattern recognition. Have you heard of a doctor's 'spidey-sense'? One Spanish study of 155 GPs showed that the 'gut feeling' of experienced practitioners was significant in detecting serious diseases (59 per cent) and was also useful in ruling out serious diseases 98 per cent of the time.[14] Lastly, and of course, most importantly, I take into account the lived experience of my patients. You are the expert on how it feels to live in your body. Listening for answers from my patients – which I could never find in a study – is one of the most important parts of providing good care.

Life is a lottery, and we cannot help where we start from. But the lessons we learn and the journey we take mean that there is always an opportunity to feel better. On various levels there is hope, for our own health now and in the future.

Doctors should feel able to empower their patients to try changes to their lifestyle and mindset as well as medical therapies to help them feel better. My hope is that this book will help you need your doctor less, and find many ways to feel better when you are not in the consulting room.

What can you expect from
Get Well, Stay Well?

In this book, I focus on six health habits that I have researched and tested with my patients in my clinic. And you don't have to take my word for it, because everything here is backed up by carefully researched evidence.

These six health habits are also free of charge. This is truly accessible and affordable health advice for everyone.

Once we have looked at the six healing health habits, we will move on to the most exciting element of the book – making it your own. I have incorporated unique templates and journal prompts that will allow you to create your own bespoke plan. Using your favourite elements from the book and journalling will help you make the practical changes you want to see in your habits, your life and your health.

How do I know this could help you? I have seen how chronic illnesses that have left my patients feeling powerless can be managed and reversed using the health habits in this book. I treat patients of all ages and suffering from all kinds of illnesses, both physical and mental.

None of this information is new or secret. It has been taught and practised for thousands of years – by a range of learned experts in various disciplines and across different cultures. A lot of this knowledge has been lost to modern medical practice, which, until relatively recently, has focused only on treating the physical body. Today, the growing body of evidence coming from controlled scientific experiments is compelling us to look again, to remember. To look after our whole health – body, mind and spirit.

How could this help you?

My patients remain my biggest inspiration and give me a huge privilege by letting me into their lives. Many of them have defied the odds and reversed chronic diseases by being open to new approaches alongside prescribed medicines.

- One elderly man was able to come off insulin and get better control of his diabetes using plant-based ready meals.
- One young solo mum was able to improve her daughter's eczema by swapping out processed meat for lentils and beans and switching cow's milk for soy milk.
- One man reversed his low-grade prostate cancer without requiring additional therapy by adopting a wholefoods, plant-based diet.
- With a single phone call, one patient was motivated enough to make changes to his life which ended years of arthritic pain and normalised his cholesterol.

The decision to change a pattern of behaviour does not just apply to physical health.

- I recall a patient who was determined to be a good dad to his teenage daughter, despite broken relationships in his past, a spinal fusion operation and chronic pain and heart disease affecting his life and decisions every day.
- I remember counselling a woman in her seventies who had finally found the strength to leave an abusive marriage.

❀ I will never forget the joy of supporting a woman in her forties who, after a lifetime of drug addiction and a traumatic history with the men in her life, was able to find love again and leave her addictions behind.

My patients have taught me a very valuable lesson over the last 20 years: the things we cannot change do not make us powerless in our lives.

On my car journey home that fateful day, I began to realise that recognising where we struggle does not mean that we cannot feel better. We can all make a shift and feel incrementally better than we did before. All it takes is a readiness to be vulnerable, and the desire to begin.

Why I'm the Plant Power Doctor

It may sound clichéd but, like most doctors, I went into my career because I wanted to help people. I chose to be a general practitioner (GP) because I love getting to know my patients, their families and the communities in which they live. Connecting with people throughout the worst of times, and helping them to imagine and work towards a time when things could feel better than they do now – that is my aim. At a time when communities and family links are becoming so rare, people come to the doctor for so much more than medical advice. They seek a friend, a confidante, a counsellor and sometimes everything in between. Patients let me into their lives and trust me, and for that, I feel hugely privileged.

Over the years I have grown to understand how wonderful – and yet how limited – the medical model can be. There are many guidelines and templates in place to 'manage' people's illnesses and, in my profession, the question of 'what' often becomes more important than 'why'.

For me, though, the question 'Why is this person suffering?' is far more important than 'What is the diagnosis?'

When I first started working as a doctor, I began to realise that people simply did not fit into the boxes we tried to put them into. The 'boxes' help us as doctors to feel confident and safe. If our patients can easily fit within diagnostic tools, we can use clear, evidence-based steps to manage their situation.

But real life is different, and people's symptoms and stories do not always fit the mould. Finding a diagnosis and treatment plan is crucial, but also noticing what patterns existed prior to that diagnosis can be highly relevant. Understanding *why* a symptom has arisen is much trickier, and is useful to think about when someone is living with a chronic disease.

- ❀ What food does a person eat?
- ❀ Who are they surrounded by?
- ❀ What do they do for a living?
- ❀ What is their social life like?
- ❀ How do they sleep at night?

Going further back sometimes helps.

- ❀ What is their relationship like with their parents?
- ❀ What infections and experiences did they have in the early years?
- ❀ Did they grow up lonely? Did they have a lot of responsibilities? Did they feel safe?

All these elements are relevant when putting the puzzle pieces of the 'why' of disease into a picture we can recognise. And sometimes we don't find a 'why'. That's okay. Moving forwards is what is most important. If we can make changes in the present that bring more happiness and health today, it will increase the chances of having more health in your life and giving more happiness to those around you in the future.

The power of plants

My journey to writing my first book, *The Plant Power Doctor*, came about by chance. My husband Richard was training to run the London Marathon, and he was getting injury after injury, with inflamed hips and ankles. Hobbling home after yet another thwarted marathon training run, he was disappointed and wanted to be well enough to do his best. He started to read about what ultrarunners do – how did they manage to run for hundreds of miles at a time? He realised that many of these runners had something in common – they ate a wholefoods, plant-based diet.[15-17]

'I'm going to give it a try,' he said to me one night. I had never looked into plant-based diets before and, to be honest, my first instinct was one of horror: 'What will our friends say? We will be social outcasts! You'll get a nutritional deficiency! How are you supposed to get enough protein?!'

Undeterred, Richard started eating more beans, rice, vegetables and fruit, and stopped eating meat, dairy, eggs, refined flour or processed foods. He started making huge progress with his training and stopped getting injured. He was training less and making better times. His inflamed ankles returned to normal. He could run a marathon before breakfast then look after the kids all day! I figured this must be some sort of coincidence, but I started looking into the medical literature.

The evidence for increasing the proportion of whole plant

foods was compelling and persuasive.[18-20] Then I felt quite embarrassed for being so sure that food had nothing to do with it. I could see the changes were really beneficial for him.

We grew up knowing that eating vegetables was a good thing, but not *how* good, and not how transformative a plant-based diet could be. Why wasn't the message being spread more widely? After six months on a wholefoods, plant-based diet, Richard ran the marathon again, an hour and ten minutes faster than his first attempt.

My own health journey

As a young doctor in a high-pressure environment, like many new physicians, I often neglected my own health. I ate too much convenience food, I often felt exhausted and my BMI was not in the healthy range. I had raised blood pressure despite being in my twenties. I wanted to feel better and have more energy to do my job. And I felt like a hypocrite. How could I tell people how to be healthier if I was not trying to be healthy myself? At the beginning of my career, I was absolutely shattered.

Having never considered the role of nutrition, I naively assumed it was a simple case of 'eat less and move more'. But how? At the time, the advice to 'cut carbs' was rife within popular culture and among my colleagues, and so I adopted a low-carb diet in an attempt to feel healthier. I was eating a lot of chicken, fish and salads.

Calorie counting ensued, and I threw myself into exercise. It worked. I lost weight, had normal blood pressure and heart rate, and I was full of energy. I felt pretty pleased with my efforts and newfound athleticism. I went from being the girl who would avoid sports at school at all costs to running half-marathons for the fun of it!

I felt that I was at optimal health. Surely this would set a benchmark for the rest of my life?

I decided to get a blood test as a way of looking at my overall health, heart disease risk, cholesterol and other proteins in the blood that carry fats (low-density lipoprotein, high-density lipoprotein, triglycerides).

I was shocked to discover that despite reducing my body fat, my blood test showed that my lipids were raised even higher. Lipids are fat-like substances found in your blood and tissues; the main one is cholesterol. Your body needs the right amounts of lipids to work normally and make hormones, but excess amounts can cause fatty deposits on the artery walls, increasing the risk of heart disease.

I have a history of heart disease in my family. My grandfather died from a heart attack at 61. My father died of a heart attack at the age of only 59. I saw my lipid numbers and I was dismayed. I felt that I would have to chalk it up to genetic destiny; if that was the hand I had been dealt, then there was nothing more I could do about it.

After my husband had the dramatic improvement with his marathon running, I wondered if there was a way to reverse my fate and take control of some of the physiological mechanisms that were raising my risk of heart disease.[21,22] I decided to go completely plant-based and monitor what this did to my blood results.

I didn't tell anyone at first. What if I found it too hard, or lost my way? But I did it. And whether it was because I had done so much research already, or just because it felt so good, it was not as challenging as I thought it would be.

A month later, I did another set of blood tests and my lipids were completely normal. I was in shock. When I turned to the literature, I could see that others had achieved similar results time and again when they adopted a wholefoods, plant-based diet.[23-25]

Why? There is very little saturated fat (which has consistently been shown in research to be the most important dietary factor), no dietary cholesterol, and abundant fibre, phytonutrients and antioxidants – all of which work together to help blood vessels become more supple and responsive – in a diet like this.[26,27]

It took that final personal experience to tip me into action, because it was then that I realised I could have some control over my genetic destiny. Although my genes loaded the gun, they did not pull the trigger. I felt I had a second chance at a long and healthy life.

I also began to think of all the families who had no idea that they could potentially have more time with the people they love – more time that I wish I had had with mine – with a few simple lifestyle changes.

Despite my story, I knew I could never base health advice for others on personal experience alone. After months of research, reviewing decades of data, it became clear that a plant-predominant eating pattern has been consistently shown to benefit human health and longevity.[28-35]

Although I have personally been thriving on a vegan lifestyle for many years, not everyone has the desire to be completely plant-based in their diet. The good news, if you are thinking this way of eating isn't for you, is that you don't have to be 100 per cent plant-based with your diet. We can see health benefits for every shift that people make towards eating more whole plant foods.

I decided to take the plunge and share some of the knowledge I had built up with my patients. It was a revelation.

I had patients whose blood pressure normalised within weeks; many were able to come off blood pressure and diabetes medications (including insulin in some with type 2 diabetes) that they had relied upon for years.

I had patients improving symptoms of endometriosis, fibroids, menopause, functional and inflammatory bowel disorders, polycystic ovarian syndrome (PCOS), diverticulosis, acne, asthma, eczema and even improvements in mood through the dietary changes they had made.

The six health habits everyone should know

'Wellness' can feel elitist, only available for those who can afford infrared saunas, expensive gym memberships, grass-fed beef and high-cost supplements. In reality, wellness is something we should all be able to get more of, whatever our budget.

My patients are not seeing me privately. They do not have an unlimited budget and many of them are in fact struggling socially and financially.

Almost every recommendation in this book is free.

I feel passionate about sharing these messages with you because, even in the worst of times, and with limited means, there are things that can help you feel better. There are also things you can do that can bring hope, or acceptance of where you are. Sometimes truly feeling these emotions is enough to begin the process of feeling better.

I should make it clear that a healthy lifestyle, therapy or a diet change is not a guaranteed cure-all. The healthiest people will still become ill and require medical care. There is an extremely import-ant role for drug therapies, surgery and evidence-based medical care to reduce long-term risk and to treat illnesses. You should never stop a prescribed medication without discussing it with your doctor. In many cases, people will still benefit from their medications.

Life is complicated and messy, with lots of factors influencing our health and ability to shift our habits. But for those of my patients who have made changes, the health transformations I have witnessed have been nothing short of extraordinary.

From those early days until now, I continue to see transformations. From young women suffering from issues such as fibroids and heavy periods to older men with issues such as chronic pain and prostate enlargement, a wholefoods, plant-based lifestyle really can make a difference. It was the reason I wrote my first book, which was the first cookbook of its kind to distil this information in an easy-to-access way. I wrote the book that I would have wanted my own family, and those I look after, to be able to read.

You are more than what you eat

Food is foundational, and we use it to make all the different parts of our bodies function properly and get the energy we need to sustain us. But it's not just about food.

Take a moment to imagine your body is a car. What you have eaten provides the car's fuel and battery. But there are other things to consider before you can drive. Do the brakes work? How's the engine sounding? Are there cracks in the window? What kind of roads will you be driving on – are there many potholes, a lot of traffic? What are the best driving conditions for your journey? Lastly, do you even know how to get where you need to be?

I have met some patients with extremely well-planned-out diets who struggle with anxiety. I have met others who exercise daily and yet burn out from lack of sleep. How we breathe, where we live, how much we move, the amount of sunlight and fresh air we feel, the things we think about, the people we surround ourselves with, the amount of time we spend laughing and hugging, the movies and TV shows we watch, the hobbies we have, the music we listen to, the social media feeds we scroll, the books we enjoy – these are the choices we make for ourselves every day that can also have profound effects on our health and happiness.

The problem is that our thoughts – whether we are ruminating on the past or worrying about the future – can keep us stuck. Our thoughts and subsequent emotions can drive our health, because they are in charge of what we do, think and feel. The things we do, think and feel dictate our daily habits and choices.

Fortunately, there are ways we can be more mindful of our emotional states, and how our habits can affect them. Importantly, our daily habits, although they may seem small, are actually crucial in engaging our body and our mind together. This book builds on the foundation research of my first book by connecting all the dots between how we live each day, as well as what we eat, to feel well. And plants still play a crucial role in providing amazing benefits – and not just when we eat them. But more on that later.

Medicine for body *and* mind *and* spirit

Medical training by necessity sometimes forces us to close our minds to the unknown. We are taught to be specific, to look for solid outcomes, and to follow the evidence base. With all this structure and security, it can make a doctor feel inadequate when someone doesn't fit the protocol. If their symptoms do not go away despite being given all the treatments that were supposed to work, we can feel stuck. So I have always tried to be open to new ideas.

When I worked in psychiatry, I learned about psychological interventions. I was taught how to perform cognitive behavioural therapy (CBT) and solution-focused brief therapy (SFBT), which could help people change their mindset.

A few years later I learned how to be a Western-style and Jikiden reiki practitioner. I have found my reiki practice incredibly useful personally and for patients struggling with pain. This is an aspect of my work I tend to talk about less, as it is often misunderstood.

Reiki is a healing technique in which a practitioner uses gentle hand movements with the intention to guide the flow of 'life force energy' through the client's body to reduce stress and promote healing. Yes, it sounds woo-woo. But it works.

Interestingly, world-leading cancer centres are now offering reiki in combination with oncological therapies as an evidence-based option for reducing pain from cancer, dealing with chemotherapy and enhancing wellbeing scores for their patients.[36,37] Several studies have now shown that reiki reduces pain in a variety of clinical settings, including for back pain, nausea, fatigue and pain relief in haemodialysis.[38-41] A meta-analysis of four randomised controlled studies into the use of reiki concluded that it produced statistically significant reductions in pain.[42] You may say, 'This is interesting, but could it just be due to the effects of a kind practitioner and some relaxing music?' Well, yes, it could. However, some studies attempt to separate these factors from the treatment itself, by comparing reiki with so-called 'sham' reiki. This is where an actor reproduces the same movements and hand positions as a trained reiki practitioner. The aim is to replicate a drug–placebo comparison, which is commonly used for pharmaceutical trials. Reiki typically shows better results than sham reiki. For example, there was a study on 45 women who had a Caesarean section, who were given either reiki or sham reiki over the incision area twice following their operation. Some women didn't receive either reiki or sham reiki, so that a comparison with no therapy could be made. Reiki produced a significant reduction in pain, blood pressure and average breathing rate compared with sham reiki and the control group. The women who received reiki also needed less pain relief.[43]

How does reiki work? So far, we don't know. As mentioned, a

connection with a practitioner, making time to relax, perhaps listening to music and engaging the parasympathetic nervous system can all play a part. But there may also be an 'energetic' explanation. Try to hold your scepticism at bay for a moment while I explain.

The aim of a reiki practitioner is not to 'heal' someone, but rather to direct energy to facilitate the person's own healing response. It is classified as a 'biofield' therapy. A biofield is simply an electromagnetic field produced by a biological organism. Getting down to a very small level, you might remember from school that the atoms in our bodies all have a nucleus made up of protons and neutrons, which is surrounded by a cloud of electrons. The positive and negative charges in the atoms of our bodies generate a small electric field, like a magnet can generate a magnetic field when you place another magnet close to it. This means each atom inside us has a tiny electrical charge. Of course, everything around us is also made from atoms, not just our bodies. Even something that looks as solid as a bed or a table is made up of atoms, and their energetic clouds of electrons. So whether you are giving someone a hug or opening a door, your electric field is pressing against the electric field of the other person or the door. You feel the push of the atoms that make up the door as something solid, but the push is electrical, not physical. The sensation you feel when you hug someone, or open a door, is actually how your brain processes the force between the two interacting energy fields. From birth, we naturally grow to recognise these sensations as physical touch. But they can really be thought of as 'energy on energy'. This energy can be used therapeutically. Studies show devices that emit pulsed electromagnetic field therapy (PEMF) can have wound-healing effects.[44] This is how I like to think about reiki: as a tool to harness electromagnetic energy in a way that promotes healing.

Another way to imagine the concept is to reflect on your own heart. How does your heart beat? It generates its own electricity. Interestingly, the electrical field of the heart is about 60 times greater in amplitude than the electric field of the brain (measured with an ECG and an EEG – electrocardiogram and electroencephalogram – respectively). The heart also has a magnetic field around 100 times larger than the brain's magnetic field. Amazingly, your heart's electromagnetic field can be detected up to a metre outside of your body (using a superconducting quantum interference device, or SQUID). Our emotional states have an impact on blood flow, stress hormones and other substances that move ions in and out of our cells. Positive states like happiness, joy, compassion or gratitude tend to extend the heart's magnetic field. Negative states like stress, anxiety, or fear tend to contract it.

The reiki practitioner is taught to provide therapy from a place of compassion, and with good intentions. I believe it is possible that the emotional state of the practitioner at the time of the therapy can also have an impact on its effectiveness for this reason. Acting from the heart seems to have more energetic potential than acting from the brain – at least when it comes to electromagnetic fields! When we understand these concepts, we begin to also understand the power of human connection and physical touch. The healing we get through a genuine hug makes much more sense when we look at the world in terms of energy transference.

If we accept the evidence presented so far that reiki could improve pain, further research into how it can be incorporated into treatment settings could be useful. However, the fact still remains that it is a financial privilege to be able to try complementary therapies at all.

Not everyone has the access, funds or indeed the inclination to delve into complementary treatments or psychological support.

So the question remained large in my mind: how could my

patients, who were time-poor, low on funds and having a hard time with their health, genuinely start to feel better?

The *Get Well, Stay Well* plan

I thought long and hard about the experiences I have had over the years, witnessing people's journeys towards health transformations. What unifying principles lie behind a state of wellness? How can emotions, beliefs and mindset facilitate healing? Lastly, how do we accept where we are in terms of health, if things are not where we want them? How do we then build a realistic future health expectation? I worked to distil those ideas down into their simplest forms, focusing on the treatment theory at the heart of every holistic and medical practice I could study. It became apparent to me that there should be a 'whole body' treatment plan that cared for a person's mind, body and emotional health – everything that makes you unique, and makes you feel well or ill. This is why I created the GLOVES framework.

In the next chapter, you will learn valuable tools that you can apply in your own life to help you stay well, or to improve your health. Sound too good to be true? It really isn't.

GLOVES

It used to surprise me to see how the smallest tweaks we make to our daily habits can accrue over time, and result in big changes to our health. Over the years, I've had patients with long-term symptoms that did not have an obvious medical explanation, such as brain fog, achy joints, chronic headaches and fatigue, who have applied the principles I share here in their own lives and were amazed at the changes they noticed. Many of them are now symptom free.

It doesn't surprise me anymore, but it is hugely gratifying to see people feeling more in control of their health. I cannot promise miracles, as I am sure you know. There are many factors in our lives that are outside of our control. This is important to recognise. We were not all born with the same advantages, and our challenges in life vary hugely. But this does not make us victims of fate either. Our own actions, thoughts and feelings are the only things we can reflect upon, and make changes to. And the results of that simple revelation can be truly remarkable.

How did I come up with the GLOVES framework? I needed a simple way to remind myself of the lifestyle habits and perspectives that were shiftable. Things that my patients could observe and change if need be. One morning in clinic I had seen a patient with a latex allergy; let's call her Millie. As a fellow healthcare professional, she had to wear gloves a lot in her work. Her skin was sore and inflamed on both hands, red raw from contact with latex gloves for hours every day. I gave her some soothing creams and emollients, and advised her to use latex-free gloves in future. She could have left at that point. That was all that was required in the consultation, and my patient, who was a nurse, would have gone away perfectly happy. But going back to the bathtub analogy, was there an underlying cause for this? A way to unblock the drain rather than just mopping the overflowing water from her bathroom floor?

I suspected there could be lifestyle factors that would reduce Millie's risk of developing other allergies, or a worsening of her contact dermatitis. She had a history of eczema, asthma and hay fever, as well as thyroid dysregulation. These are all conditions that can be caused by an overactive immune response to environmental triggers. We talked about her life in general. I often find it really helpful to ask my patients about what a typical day looks like for them.

Remember, it is our daily habits that will accrue to make a lifestyle.

It turns out she had been feeling anxious of late, and was so busy with work that she'd often grab foods on the go without giving herself time to digest them. Millie would drink a coffee and croissant on the way to work. Then, for lunch, she'd buy a ham and cheese sandwich, a cola and a chocolate bar from the canteen each day to keep her energy levels up, then suffer bloating and exhaustion later in the day. Too tired to cook when she got home, she'd eat a takeaway and stay up scrolling on her phone to help her wind down before the next day began. Other than rushing around the ward, she did not exercise and rarely went outside. She liked to party on her days off, but she had been struggling to focus at work despite cutting down on alcohol. Millie lived in a flat share. This was a typical day for her. She decided after our consultation that she'd make three small shifts. She agreed to spend Sundays cooking two meals that she could keep in the fridge or freezer for the week ahead. She'd make the time to eat breakfast and lunch while sitting, and just notice the food she was eating. Lastly, she decided to prioritise a good sleep routine by waking up the same time of day all week and getting to bed an hour earlier than she normally would. These three simple shifts felt manageable to her, and she agreed to them before she left.

When I saw Millie again three months later, her asthma had improved dramatically, she no longer had dry skin, and she was able to come off her antihistamines and steroid creams. She had also been able to reduce her inhaler use and stop one of them completely. I did not tell her this would happen (I obviously couldn't know for sure), and yet she was thrilled with the unexpected shifts that she had noticed with just a few small tweaks to her routine. I realised that in her case, taking off the latex gloves was obviously important for her eczema, but that by eliminating some of the underlying causes of her skin issues, she was also 'taking off the gloves' figuratively, getting down into the root causes, and reaping the rewards.

In clinic I use gloves a lot. For all intimate examinations, for many procedures and for infection control, my box of gloves is always handy. I realised after I saw Millie, and after I had taken off yet another pair of gloves after a consultation that day, that the letters in 'GLOVES' perfectly aligned with the factors I believe have the biggest impact on our long-term health – the factors that we have some control over.

When you hear what each of the words in the GLOVES framework stands for, you may roll your eyes.

Gratitude
Love
Outside
Vegetables
Exercise
Sleep

You may find it strange that a medical doctor is talking about emotions and how they impact the body. But I have seen from 20 years of clinical practice that in *every one* of my patients with chronic diseases, emotional regulation can play a pivotal role in the quality of their life, the severity of their symptoms and the speed of progression of their diseases. Thankfully, I am not the only voice advocating for a whole-body understanding of our health – the research is stacking up and is increasingly compelling.

Canadian physician and researcher Dr Gabor Maté has written about the link between the mind and body in a number of books, and his research has focused on the connection between stress and disease.[45]

US-based psychiatrist Bessel van der Kolk, author of *The Body Keeps the Score*, has spent his career researching the impact of trauma on the body.[46]

Scottish kindness scientist Dr David Hamilton has written extensively about how people can harness their mind and emotions to improve their mental and physical health.[47]

Cognitive scientist Dr Scott Barry Kaufman drew on the work of psychologists such as Abraham Maslow to help us discover new ways to grow and explore human potential through his research. He created a beautiful analogy that the human experience is like a sailboat. With holes in the hull of your sailboat, you can't go anywhere – all physical and mental energy is spent in trying to make sure all of the holes are plugged: physical safety, health, self-esteem.

The sail of the boat in the analogy represents purpose, love and exploration. In order to grow, you have to open up the sail and be vulnerable to all the wind and waves that life brings.[48]

Neurobiologist Gina Rippon pioneered our understanding of neuroplasticity and brain function, as well as helping us to see how a sense of belonging affects our brains and bodies.[49]

You might also be aware of the importance of gut health on wellbeing, and how research teams at the American Gut Project and King's College London show us more about the exciting connection between the microbes within us and many aspects of our wellness – including our mental health and immune function. I talked about this in my first book too.

Thanks to these brilliant and brave pioneers, along with many others, we are talking more about the mind and body connection. But most doctors do not feel confident enough to incorporate these findings into their treatment plans and make available a whole-body care plan for everyone.

Physical symptoms are proven to affect our mental health, and our mental health is proven to affect our perception of how our bodies feel, and how physical symptoms of illness feel. More than this, changing our physiology is a powerful way of reaching the emotional brain in a way that our logical mind is unable to do. We can't just tell our brains to 'calm down' when we are feeling overwhelmed or stressed. But when we express our emotions physically, through movement such as therapeutic breathing, yoga, running, weights, dance or tai chi, for example, we can shift our physical state. This has an almost immediate knock-on effect on our mental state too. I'll explain more as we go through each of the GLOVES components in turn, helping you understand the impact of these factors in a practical and science-backed way.

Use the framework I have set out in this book to decide which tools can be most easily introduced into your daily life. We are all different, with a variety of life experiences and challenges that are unique to us. Some of the areas of my framework you'll have already integrated into your life without realising, while others may need looking at.

Remember, you are the expert in your own body and mind, but please be open to finding a health habit to try from the framework, even if it feels silly or strange at first. You'll read certain parts of this book and they will make sense to you, while others you may initially reject or feel are not for you. If you feel strongly that something is not for you, I'd urge you to spend a moment reflecting on this. Sometimes we have a strong emotional reaction to the things that 'hit a nerve', and these can be the areas we struggle with the most. What you will read are a variety of evidence-based tips and tools that you can use if you want to.

Keep reading to understand the benefits of all the habits I talk about in the GLOVES framework. There is a table called 'GLOVES daily actions guide' on page 281 that gives you a summary of all the practical tips and exercises that are mentioned. Use the table if you need an easy reference guide for the exercises you'll want to add to your personalised plan later in the book. I want you to treat this book like a friendly support that you come back to, as your life evolves and your needs change. Keep it by your bedside table, in your bag or on your coffee table. Write in the margins of it, dog-ear the pages and scribble notes. If the book is lived in, I'll know you have enjoyed using it!

Healthy for you *and* healthy for the planet

Eco-anxiety is a growing concern. Does this affect you? When I reflect on wider concerns beyond human health, such as planetary health and the climate crisis, I see that we are one small part of a larger ecosystem. Our health and the health of the planet are connected. We live in a world overrun with plastics, and ocean plastics largely originate from abandoned fishing nets.[50] Epidemic disease risks are rising, largely from breeding increasing amounts of poultry in cramped conditions.[51] Antibiotic-resistant infections are also on the rise, driven primarily by having to give antibiotics to animals that are bred in factory farms.[52] Our waterways are being polluted from silage runoffs, which impact rivers and cause damaging algal blooms and dead zones in our oceans.[53] We are losing many wild spaces and species of animals due to deforestation, largely driven by the cattle industry.[54]

Environmental scientists are clear that animal agriculture, as we know it, is responsible for a significant proportion of the problems we, as a species and as a planet, are having to deal with.[55]

The natural world is struggling with health issues in just the same ways as we are.

One solution to help us and the planet at the same time is a plant-predominant diet. Research shows that this way of eating is good for us and that it creates a more sustainable world.[56]

What helps the individual also helps the community, while also taking pressure off the planetary ecosystems that sustain us. This is a win-win for everyone.

We have seen that prejudice, pain and chronic illness can really impact the life chances and lives of a whole generation of people. When we add the climate crisis, the rising cost of living and increasing social disconnection to the picture, it is clear we need to change course.

It is my sincere hope that this book will provide a way for you to connect some of the missing dots in your life and achieve more health, more happiness and ultimately contribute more healing to the people around you and to the world at large.

This book is a simple science-based guide to create a bespoke health toolkit just for you. It is your blueprint for life, so go ahead and make it your own. If you haven't done it yet, go and grab a pen and start writing notes in the margin (yes, it's okay to scribble in this book!). You can come back to your favourite parts as often as you need to.

The *Get Well, Stay Well* plan in the final chapter of the book is all about you. It can be adapted over time as your health and happiness goals change. Don't worry, I'll take you by the hand and guide you through the process step by step. Just remember to keep the book handy somewhere you can see it – by your bed or on your desk – so you can write thoughts and ideas in it as they come up, and refer back to it as often as you need to.

Let's dive in!

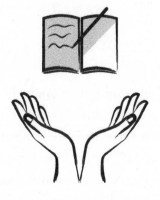

Gratitude

Y ou will notice that I place gratitude and love, two emotional states, as the first steps to a healthy body and mind. This is not simply because they are the first two letters of the 'GLOVES' framework. They are fundamental to our wellbeing.

I know that it is almost impossible to feel grateful for unwanted things. It is also very hard to feel grateful for unfair things. The truth of living is that we will all experience hard and unfair things – and some of us more than others. Death, disappointment and disasters are a fundamental part of living. Figuring out how to live *with* our feelings, *learn* from them and move *through* them is one of the biggest struggles in life. Feeling good is not a guarantee, but for most of us, it is a by-product of knowing a little bit more about how we tick and who we are.

I realised at a young age that sometimes the people I loved the most were struggling no matter how much I loved them. As a doctor, I also saw that sometimes the traumas and life experiences of my patients were too overwhelming, too tragic, to forget. I understand that no matter how much insight we develop, the rational brain is often left feeling helpless. But you are not helpless. Even in the worst of times.

I had a patient a few years ago, let's call her Nicola, who received a terminal cancer diagnosis. She was in her mid-thirties with two young children, and many hopes and dreams. Suddenly, her world felt shattered. The worst part for her was knowing she would not be able to be present for her children as they grew up. Despite this heartbreaking situation, whenever I consulted with her, she had an air of calmness to her. There were tears at times, and moments of overwhelm while she processed the journey and what plans she had to make. But the overall feeling I got from her was one of acceptance. Time and again I have counselled patients in whom fear, anxiety and anger were understandably the main emotional states they described feeling. When I asked Nicola about it, she simply said: 'I have had my time. It was less time than I wanted. But it was so full of joy. Why waste what I have left with misery? I want my children to remember me like this. I want my legacy to be for my children to know that love is all there is. And I love them. Their father loves them. And when I am gone, they can love each other and remember that I will see them again. And for that, I feel genuinely grateful.' The wisdom of her words always stayed with me. She died several months later, but I know that in those weeks and months she had the chance to make some special memories for her family. There was healing among the pain. There was genuine gratitude for a life lived to the full. I believe it was her feeling of gratitude that allowed Nicola to die peacefully, and brought some comfort to her family after she was gone. For Nicola, the choice of gratitude did not change her diagnosis, but it allowed her to die how she wanted, and I also believe it helped her children process the pain of her loss in a different way.

How gratitude affects your health

The limbic system is the part of the brain responsible for emotional experiences, and it includes the thalamus, hippocampus, amygdala, cingulate gyrus, and hypothalamus. The hypothalamus is responsible for regulating bodily functions, including hunger, sleep, metabolism and how we grow. Studies have shown that gratitude activates the whole limbic system and in particular the hypothalamus, making these systems function more effectively.[1-3]

Numerous studies have linked gratitude to better sleep; it not only increases the quality and duration of our sleep, but also decreases the time it takes to fall asleep.[4,5]

One of the brain's responses to gratitude is to activate its reward centre, flooding our brains with the feel-good chemicals dopamine and serotonin. This starts a cycle in our minds and reflects how we think about and see the world. Showing gratitude has been linked to decreased pain levels, lower blood pressure and a reduction in stress levels.[6-8]

Gratitude is not just effective for people with good mental health. One study took almost 300 adults, many of whom were college students who were seeking mental health counselling. On average, they reported low levels of mental health, and struggled with depression and anxiety. They were split into three groups: the first group wrote letters of gratitude for three weeks, the second group wrote down their thoughts and feelings about negative experiences, and the third group did not do any writing, and underwent psychotherapy alone. What was the outcome?

The people who wrote gratitude letters reported significantly better mental health after four weeks, as well as 12 weeks after their writing exercise ended.[9] The creative writing group (writing about their feelings) and the psychotherapy group both experienced less of an improvement. This suggests that not only is gratitude effective for people who are struggling with their mental health, but that gratitude practices alongside counselling could have a big impact.

We all know that negative emotions, like boredom and stress, can make us dive straight into the biscuit tin. This is why it is interesting to note that one study even showed that practising feeling gratitude can help young people eat better. When the participants practised feeling gratitude every day, it was found that they were much more likely to make better food choices.[10] Gratitude research has consistently shown that thankful people also have higher energy levels, are more creative and are generally healthier.[11] It packs a powerful punch, not just for our minds but also for our bodies.

When we are open-minded to finding these two key emotional states of gratitude and love, and introduce health habits that actively encourage them, we can notice more easily when we feel grateful, loving or loved.[12] We can hold on to them more often. When we can understand better what makes us feel gratitude and love, we can also start seeking more of it. In this way, we can spend more time in a positive emotional state. Have you ever noticed that when you're having a bad day, you start to notice more and more things that are going wrong? Similarly, when you're thinking of buying a new car, and you suddenly start seeing the car you have been researching on every road you pass? What we focus on impacts what we see. It sounds obvious, but it is seldom recognised that we can use these emotions as anchors when we experience life's ups and downs, as well as actively seeking them out to pre-empt or navigate times of stress.

Research shows that our emotions affect the way we function physically and mentally, even if we are unaware and the emotions are underlying.[13] This means that sometimes the body gives signals *first*, before we can work out the emotion that could be impacting how we feel.[14]

Let me give you a simple example of how I use one gratitude health habit in my practice to help treat my patients.

Jay, one of my patients, was suffering from headaches. He was adamant he was not stressed and that nothing was on his mind. He had a great job he enjoyed, healthy friendships and marriage, and was delighted to have had a baby boy a few months ago. Jay was a regular gym-goer and felt his life was going in the right direction. We had ruled out serious symptoms and signs, and we were left with the diagnosis of 'tension headache'.

Painkillers are the mainstay of treatment, but why were these headaches happening? Probing further into his relationships, he shared that he had not spoken to his father in over a year and was feeling a lot of regret over the loss of the relationship, and that of a grandfather figure for his baby son. It transpired that this was probably the underlying reason why he was drinking a few more beers than he wanted each night, and was struggling to get to sleep.

We talked through a variety of ways he could find peace in the situation he was in. Jay felt clear that he did not want to re-establish contact with his father. But he did want to experience peace around this decision. We went through some options and he decided to try a form of journalling. I call this exercise the 'meaning maker'. I advised Jay to write down the facts in his relationship with his father as they stood, without judging them to be 'good' or 'bad', 'right' or 'wrong'. We discussed that writing the facts of what happened, rather than focusing on the way he felt about those facts, was a tool to help separate him from an immediate emotional response each time he thought about what happened between them.

In Jay's case, he wrote, 'My father did not tell me the truth about his finances' and 'My father asked me to lend him money', rather than writing 'My father used me', 'My father betrayed me' or 'My father thinks I am a fool'.

This simple exercise in itself gave Jay the space to decide what meaning he wanted to make from the facts.

The second step in this exercise for him was to write down some of the ways in which he felt grateful for the lessons his father had taught him – including the unwanted lessons. Jay wrote: 'I am grateful I had the chance to show up with integrity. I am grateful I could see how a lack of honesty impacts my relationships' and 'I am grateful for all the ways my father helped me learn the value of nurturing people in my life'.

The next day, Jay decided to write a letter to his dad. It was a letter of forgiveness and acceptance of who he was. He did not want his dad in his life at that time and felt no need to send the letter. But the act of simply writing the letter was powerfully cathartic. Jay also decided to try a daily breathing exercise. When I saw him a few weeks later, Jay's headaches had resolved.

I have witnessed the power of the 'meaning-maker' exercise many times. I have honestly seen it completely change how my patients perceive relationships and experiences, helping them process a sense of victimhood and resentments that some have held for years – and by doing so, treating an underlying root cause of a physical, mental or emotional health issue they hadn't been able to shift.

The 'meaning maker' allows you to make a meaning about the events of your life that serves you. It is a useful tool when thinking about a specific person, event or situation. Take a moment to do one of the breathing techniques from page 240 for 60 seconds before thinking about this.

'Meaning-maker' exercise

Firstly, write down the details of a situation that you feel angry, upset about or hurt by. You can write it however you want to, explaining why it bothered you.

Now, write down the facts of the situation, and include nothing about how you feel, what you think the situation means or your opinions of the person or event. Try to avoid emotive language like 'neglected', 'gossiped', 'betrayed', 'cheated', 'heartbroken', 'painful', 'abandoned' or 'unfair'. Just write the bare facts of the event.

> Look at the facts for a moment. What meaning would you like to give this event in your life moving forwards? What do you feel this event taught you? What parts of yourself do you like more since this event? Are there parts of yourself that you are proud of, having been through this experience?
>
> What could you be grateful for, that you now know since this experience?
>
> I am grateful that . . .
>
> If you want to, you could use this 'meaning-maker' prompt to write a forgiveness letter (page 89). The letter will be for yourself. But sometimes, if it feels like it will benefit the other person, forgiveness letters can also be sent.

A formula for happiness

The evolutionary function of anxiety, fear or anger is easier to see; when triggered by a threat, we can prepare to fight or flee. But the evolutionary advantages of positive emotions are arguably more subtle. Research has shown that positive feelings such as love, awe, joy and amusement can help to expand our awareness.[15] Brain imaging even shows that positive emotions can expand our peripheral vision, so we can more literally begin to 'see the wood for the trees'.[16] This expanded perspective helps us to make discoveries, form friendships and acquire skills – showing that we need happiness on an evolutionary level, not only to live a more fulfilling life, but also to improve our overall chances of long-term survival.

The connection between health and happiness is a two-way street. People with positive attitudes tend to move more, tend not to smoke, have stronger immune systems, eat better foods, wear their seatbelts, drink in moderation and reach out to their community.

There is actually a World Database of Happiness,[17] collecting thousands of studies examining 'subjective happiness scores' from every angle of life. People in countries affected by war, poverty and disease tend to be at the bottom of the rankings. Scores will only begin to creep up once things like basic healthcare and personal freedom to make decisions are taken care of, and people can find more time in their day for laughter than for anger, worry or sadness. Prosperity can have a big impact on happiness, of course, but so does culture and comparison.

A painful truth is that often the things we think will make us happy are just plain wrong. The job with better pay, the better-looking partner, the bigger mortgage to pay for a bigger house or car: all of these assumptions are unreliable.

Researcher Dan Buettner wrote *The Blue Zones of Happiness*,[18] having delved into the happiness research and the lessons he could learn from the world's most content people. He came up with a blueprint for happiness, which was encompassed by three key words: 'pleasure' (feeling happy), 'purpose' (life goals) and 'pride' (life satisfaction). He also distilled what is needed for a happy life in his 'Power 9' tool, which includes: a romantic partner, community, friends, to be likeable, to move your body, to get plenty of sleep, to live and work in an environment that supports your needs, to set goals and look forward, to choose to live in a happy place. I urge you to read his book to understand the tools I have paraphrased here. What struck me most about Dan's work was that despite much in the self-development literature focusing on the self, it's actually when you focus on community, and cultivate a life where you can work close to where you live, make friends in your community and share your life with people you love, that most happiness can be found. When I read Dan's book and some of the studies in the database, it helped me to refocus my own GLOVES formula in a way that some of these basic tenets of wellbeing could be addressed. Thankfulness, love, exercise, nature, sleep and purpose all came up time and again as ways to live a longer and more fulfilled life.[19]

How can I feel grateful when I am in pain?

Pain is one of the universal experiences of being alive. We all experience it, physically and emotionally. The problem is, we are much more vulnerable to the negative effects of pain when we try to push it away.

A patient once told me he tried to ignore his debts by taking comfort in drinking alcohol and gambling, because he only wanted to be happy. That short-term hit was a wonderful distraction from the situation he needed to face. But in doing this, he was not only worsening his debt but also damaging his health. This is a tendency we are all prone to and it can take many forms: social media scrolling, shopping, porn, alcohol, biscuits, and binge-watching TV shows, to name a few! The short-term dopamine hit is a great way to distract us from asking ourselves the 'Big Questions' or addressing the things that cause us pain in our lives. Watching a great TV series can itself be a joyful and inspiring experience, as can having a glass of wine with friends. But a habit becomes less helpful for us if we are doing it to distract from discomfort on a consistent basis.

I see many patients having to living with chronic pain conditions. For example, my autistic patients and those with fibromyalgia also have to deal with heightened physical pain sensations, which can link to higher rates of depression and anxiety.[20-24] Although these mechanisms are complex, we do see evidence that positive emotions can reduce pain perception and so are a valuable tool when dealing with pain.[25] A study conducted to evaluate the effect of gratitude on pain indicated that 16 per cent of the subjects in the study who kept a gratitude journal reported reduced pain.[26] By regulating the level of dopamine, gratitude reduces subjective feelings of pain.

Pain comes from the same place in our brains as pleasure.[27] In facing and acknowledging that we feel pain – sadness, fear, anger – we can start the process of finding gratitude again. Becoming numb does not make us happy, because it also numbs the joy.

For a lot of us, gratitude does not come easily and that's completely normal. As humans, we tend to have a negativity bias, meaning that even when positive and negative experiences are of equal intensity, negative experiences are hardwired to have a more potent effect on our emotions and thoughts.[28] This is said to provide an evolutionary advantage, as it is more critical for survival to avoid a harmful stimulus than to pursue a potentially helpful one. But as previously stated, there are also long-term advantages to positive emotional states. Positive emotions can improve recovery from illness and may even improve chances of survival in the long term.[29,30]

Choosing to make time for gratitude habits, even during times of great pain, is your conscious way to take some control back, proactively offsetting any negativity bias and allowing you to feel more alive.

How often do we spare a moment to think about what we are enjoying and loving about our lives at this very moment? This is something we can purposely do to reap life's biggest rewards.

Simple habits that encourage gratitude

Regular bedtimes

Although research tells us grateful thoughts can help you get a good night's sleep, ensuring you focus on regularity with bedtimes will also reduce your risk of anxiety and make room for positive emotional states.[15] For more on the power of sleep, head to page 255.

Going out in nature consistently

We will understand more about the power of nature in the Outside section on page 103, but it is worth adding here that noticing what's beautiful in nature is one of the key elements of what makes mindfulness such a valuable mental health tool.[16] Noticing the shapes of the leaves, birdsong, trees in the distance or even how the air feels different are ways to cultivate 'an attitude of gratitude' on a normal day.

Bedtime exercise

Think of three things you are grateful for in bed, as you wake up, or as you fall asleep. This can start the day and finish it with a sense that you are noticing and appreciating more of the good in your routines.

A gratitude journal

One of the most popular gratitude exercises is a gratitude journal. Keep a journal on your bedside table and every evening, spend a few minutes writing down the things that you are grateful for. On the not-so-great-days, look back over previous days' entries to boost your mood.

Saying 'thank you'

Tell other people at work or home 'thank you' when they have done something kind for you, no matter how small. Observe how the good feelings ripple outwards.

Go back to the old days of writing letters and take time out to send a handwritten note to someone, thanking them for something or just to say you are thinking of them.

Aim to speak to someone (in person or online) with the purpose of giving them real thanks. It could be a positive restaurant review, or a thank you to the barista at your local coffee house. It could be a mum at school pick-up or a cashier at the supermarket. It could be an inspirational post online.

Photo log

Take pictures of the things that you love and that make you smile. This could be anything, from your children or grandchildren to the birds that sit outside your window. Return to this album on low days.

A gratitude jar

This is a lovely way to remind yourself of all the positive moments (especially if started on the first of a month and reviewed at the end, or even a new year's jar to be opened and looked at on the following New Year's Eve!). Just get some paper or a sticky note and write one thing you are grateful for each day. Fold it and put it into the jar. This is a fun way for kids to reframe their experiences too.

Pay someone a compliment every day

I try to find something I admire about every patient I see. We all have special qualities, and highlighting these will make us and other people feel better.

A thanks-giving meal

Could you share something that you are grateful for with your family? If not daily, then once a week?

Which of these would you like to try? Write one of them in your journal.

Your journal prompts

If you have a meditation practice, journalling shortly afterwards can be helpful, as any thoughts or preoccupations that have naturally bubbled to the surface of your mind can be written down. This allows you to either process what you were thinking about or create a plan around how to tackle anything that might come up.

1. Thought-dump (as above).
2. List things you are grateful for, such as health, relationships, opportunities or things that have happened or that you are looking forward to.
3. List some of the things you want to focus more on in life, or things you hope to achieve or the person you'd like to be. Doing this in the present tense – 'I am . . .' (see visualisation section on page 56) – can help you to engage your emotions in a more tangible way, and allows your body to know how it might feel to realise these goals.

Loss and heartbreak

I have seen time and again with my patients experiencing huge challenges, including ill health, grief and emotional and physically debilitating pain, that they can still find gratitude, and once they do, it helps them move forward and feel better.

Your loss may be recent and all you want to do is lie in bed listening to sad songs, or it may be that you are many weeks, months or even years after the loss and feel embarrassed to talk to people about it, as you 'should be over it by now'. Remember that your emotions need time and space to heal, just as a broken bone does. A plaster cast protects your bone as it fuses back together – no one expects you to run a marathon just after you had a plaster cast applied to your leg. The same is true for emotional injury.

Remember, the feeling of rejection follows the same pathway

in the brain as physical pain, and the same chemicals are released as in withdrawal from addiction. You are not 'imagining' the pain. Heartbreak literally hurts. Your emotions need the same attention and care as broken bones do.

Tools for navigating loss and heartbreak

'Feel the feelings' exercise

Noticing the emotions and letting them pass through you is important. Be that grief (over the loss and what it represented to you), confusion ('Who am I without this projected future?'), sadness (the loss of something or someone loved in death or heartbreak), anger ('How could they do this to me?'), hope ('Maybe we will get back together'), shame ('It's my fault' or 'I could have done more' or 'There's something wrong with me'). All emotions are valid. They may not all reflect objective reality, but noticing them in the first instance, and allowing them space is important. See if you can allow yourself a moment each day to accept what emotions are coming up for you, and recognise how they shape your actions and reactions.

'A week of you' exercise

Do something for yourself every day — a brisk walk, a call with a friend, a massage, a yoga class, one lovely meal. Something that reminds you that you have no choice but to continue to live, and truly appreciate yourself in this new reality. Learning something new like pottery, writing or art can concentrate your focus and take you out of your thoughts for a while, and is also a good way to meet new people and boost your confidence.

Tips for working through grief

- ❀ **Breathe to release grief.** When you are ready, try some of the breathing exercises on page 240.
- ❀ **It's good to talk.** We will all grieve. And yet many in society are uncomfortable with conversations about the end of relationships and the end of life. Being the kind of person that is willing to talk to others about that process – with an understanding that grief rarely goes away as much as ebbs and flows – helps other people to feel less alone. I do believe we need more conversations about grief. Silence and avoidance ultimately hurt us, and can magnify feelings of loneliness.
- ❀ **Let it be.** Let go of expectations – for yourself and others. In the case of grief, that usually means letting go of expectations of family or friends – or even of yourself – to do certain things or feel better by a certain time. In the case of a relationship break-up, do not stalk them online, reach out to fill the empty feeling ('drunk dial' or otherwise) or focus your attention on making them feel a certain way.

Emotional tie-cutting exercise

Buddha is reported to have said that the root of all suffering lies in attachment. Attachment can be to people, things or outcomes. It can even be to our identity and our existing thought patterns. Like the four seasons come and go, there comes a time to let go of certain ways of acting and reacting. Emotional tie-cutting (also known as cord-cutting) is a psychological technique that spans secular and spiritual traditions. Although it has no scientific basis, it is really a form of visualisation, which has been shown to be beneficial. The aim is to compassionately cut the emotional ties you have with someone, to ease the process of moving forward. It is most useful when you are thinking of someone with negativity, or perhaps romantically preoccupied with someone who does not feel the same way. Doing the exercise does not necessarily mean you will have no further contact with the person – this is not an option for many people when relationships end, especially those with shared children. It simply allows space for a new way of interacting. The exercise can be done with relationships that are ongoing. In a marriage or a parent–child relationship, it can create the space for new levels of connection, and can add fresh perspectives. It can also be useful for seemingly trivial interactions (for example, coworkers, or people in our lives who 'push our buttons'). It can provide the space for us to detach, and see them in a different light.

There are various ways to do the exercise, but I chose to create a simple statement that can be said out loud, with compassion.

Sitting somewhere peaceful, say (out loud):

'Whatever is yours, I return to you.
Whatever is mine, I return to me.
I release you with love.'

As you say the words, visualise threads connecting the two of you and imagine gently cutting them away.

It is very simple but surprisingly effective. Remember this exercise can also be done with belief systems. If you want to change a feeling about yourself, your limiting beliefs or perhaps your perception of people in general, give it a try and see how it changes your state of mind.

A philosophy to consider when grieving

Grief is not a problem to be fixed, and platitudes won't bring our loved ones back. The wound left by loss cannot be erased; after all, we don't want to forget the person or 'move on'. We want to still feel some connection to them, and recognise the importance they had in our lives.

We have to adjust to living with the wound. We have to keep going, to process and live with the pain and despair as we adjust to a different life without that person.

Therapy or counselling is great at times like this because it allows us to speak to someone objective who won't try to minimise our experience and will provide us a safe place to experience the raw emotions we are feeling. If you are in a position to be offered complementary grief or bereavement therapy (some hospices and community counselling services do this, for example), I urge you to be brave and try it. It might feel silly at first, but talking out loud has been proven to offer huge healing benefits – particularly in cases where you might not have family or friends to listen. If you don't feel comfortable with the therapist, you can ask to try another one. Don't give up straight away.

Being with others who remember the person and talking about the lost loved one can also bring some comfort, if that option is available to you.

Gradually, as we grow around our wounds, we can remember someone without the acute burden of pain.

There is a centuries-old Japanese repair technique called *kintsugi*, which means 'golden repair' or 'joining with gold'. When pottery is broken, rather than discard it, or hide the cracks, the repairer fills the gaps with lacquer dusted with or mixed with powdered gold, silver or platinum – which tells and celebrates the object's life story, and makes the object even more beautiful and valuable. (The practice aligns with Zen Buddhist beliefs around the beauty of imperfect things and being mindful of wastefulness.)

How is this relevant for you? Don't try to suppress or ignore your pain, mask it with other things or hide it from others. It will not go away. Doing this could make you quite ill. Grief and heartbreak mean that you loved and were loved, and that is beautiful.

Think about some of the ways you can begin to process your pain with some of the exercises in this book. Bringing meaning to your experiences can be a helpful way to come to a place of acceptance of what is. Through this process, you will create your very own repair with 'gold' – something beautiful on the inside and out.

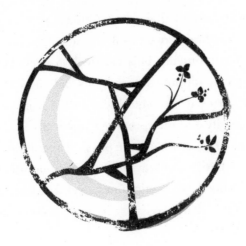

Trauma and the body, mind and emotions

Emotions give us physical sensations (e.g. butterflies in your stomach) and are revealed in our facial expressions and body language. In turn, physical sensations can impact our emotions – a soft, warm breeze or the sun on our backs might put us at ease, while loud, clanging noises can put us on edge. Experiencing trauma can put this normal feedback loop out of sync, and can cause a host of physical symptoms.

'Trauma' has become a broad term that is often used in conversations and on social media, but is seldom understood. I think psychiatrist Bessel van der Kolk, author of *The Body Keeps the Score*, describes it best. He wrote about the idea of how trauma can 'live' within us, not just within our thoughts. He explains that 'trauma' can stem from a one-time event or an ongoing experience – from a car accident to wartime combat – and can cause a lifetime of flashbacks, nightmares, isolation, insomnia, hypervigilance, rage and even physical illness.

Brain scans reveal that when trauma patients experience flashbacks, their brains react as if the actual trauma were happening in that moment. This can feel so overwhelming that survivors cope by suppressing emotions and physical sensations. As a result, they can become disconnected from their bodies, unable to identify and interpret their physical sensations. When you can't understand what your physical sensations are telling you, the body finds other ways to demand your attention: many trauma survivors develop migraines, neck and back pain, fibromyalgia, asthma, digestive issues, irritable bowel syndrome and chronic fatigue.

Our bodies 'store' experiences – good and bad – and this can increase the likelihood of physical ailments in surprising ways. I had a patient who came to see me, having been discharged from hospital recently. He had been stabbed by a stranger in a high-rise apartment block, and following the unprovoked attack, he could not walk up the stairs of his own apartment block without experiencing visceral flashbacks to the moment of his attack. He also developed severe digestive issues and chronic unexplained chest pains in the months that followed.

Thankfully, most of us will not go through something so obviously traumatic. We are not always aware of the effects of cumulative 'mini-stressors' in life that can also precipitate anxiety or physical sensations. Many of my patients have had debilitating panic attacks 'out of the blue' and cannot think of an underlying reason. Fortunately, there are ways to approach these symptoms, without unhealthy 'navel-gazing', and with the aim of alleviating physical symptoms.

Your parasympathetic nervous system can calm your physical body, which includes your brain. And so, in a stealth way, some physical therapies can calm your mind too. Studies have shown practices such as yoga really can help people deal with the symptoms of post-traumatic stress.[31] Eye movement desensitisation and reprocessing therapy (EMDR), in which a trained therapist will guide you to think about a trauma while moving your eyes back and forth, left to right, can do the same thing.[32] Sometimes physical interventions can help the brain reprocess the memories so that they no longer cause as much emotional pain.

Free things you can try that activate the parasympathetic nervous system in the same way include breathing exercises, therapeutic dance, music, cold-water therapy and, of course, meditation. If you already do some of these things and feel they are making a difference but wondered if that was simply the placebo effect at work: the answer is no! They *are* doing you good.

When dealing with trauma, I can't emphasise enough the importance of speaking to a qualified psychologist, psychiatrist or counsellor. This is a proven, hugely important and integral step towards healing.

Please also try some of the gratitude health habits here and see how they impact the way you feel each day. Below is a wonderful exercise which combines a simple physical intervention with a positive phrase. It is an evidence-based treatment for PTSD as well as other mental health conditions. I'm excited for you to try it!

Tapping exercise (EFT)

Emotional freedom technique (EFT) is an effective body-tapping technique used to treat stress, anxiety and depression.[33] It is a body-centred therapy like yoga, massage, tai chi, qigong and acupuncture. EFT was developed by author Gary Craig in the 1990s, based on his study of work done by Roger Callahan in thought field therapy (TFT). The two components of EFT are gentle tapping on the energy lines, or meridians, used in acupuncture and acupressure, combined with current psychotherapy scripts or CBT. It has been well researched, and is a simple tool you can learn to do on yourself.

What I love about it most is that it's easy to use, it is free and you can do it any time. A practitioner can provide in-depth help if needed.

1. Begin by saying what is on your mind; it could be a phys-ical pain, a fear or perhaps something you are angry about. Rate your negative emotion on a scale of 0 to 10.

2. Say something positive about yourself, which identifies the issue and includes a statement of acceptance. For example: 'Even though I have this pain, I love and accept myself.'

3. You might never have done this before and it might sound self-indulgent and uncomfortable. But please give it a try.

4. Use your fingers to tap around seven to nine times on each area marked in the illustration opposite.

5. As you tap, say your chosen phrase.

Tapping procedures can differ slightly between experts, but most incorporate these locations:

❀ the heel of the hand
❀ three areas around the eye
❀ the area below the nose
❀ the area below the lips
❀ the collarbone

❋ the underarm
❋ the top of the head.

Repeat roughly seven to nine taps on each spot.

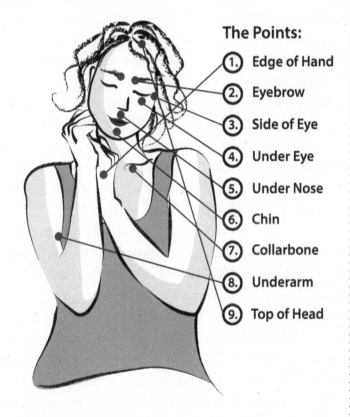

The Points:

1. Edge of Hand
2. Eyebrow
3. Side of Eye
4. Under Eye
5. Under Nose
6. Chin
7. Collarbone
8. Underarm
9. Top of Head

How do you feel? You can repeat the cycle as many times as you need to feel calmer and more positive.

I recommend both adults and children try this. Wonderfully, more and more schools are bringing mental health habits like tapping into the classroom, which is a really helpful way to aid children in learning more about emotional regulation.

How your imagination can improve your health

You might have heard of visualisation. You might have heard of manifestation. What on earth are these terms – is this all woo-woo nonsense? No, it's not.

If you can't imagine a positive future, how are you going to see the signposts to help you get there?

The power of our imagination should not be underestimated. Many professional athletes use visualisation techniques to excel at their sports, and research shows that if people imagine themselves performing well in a task, they do better – without physically doing anything different.[34] The imagination can inspire motivation, improved concentration and greater confidence.[35,36]

Many studies show the power of the imagination, or mental rehearsal, on muscle strength.[34,37] In one of the studies, the subjects were asked to imagine themselves flexing their arm muscles as hard as they could for 15 minutes, 5 days a week, for 12 weeks. The first group were told to do this as though they were watching themselves (like in a movie), the second were told to imagine themselves within their bodies in real time (as though they were doing the exercise now) and the third group didn't imagine anything.

The third group (the control group) and the first group showed no changes in their muscle strength, but the second group, who imagined themselves in real time, showed a 10.8 per cent increase in muscle strength without having done any exercise at all![37] Like a *mental rehearsal* for real life, the practice paid off. The technique of imagining yourself achieving physical goals is also invaluable for rehabilitation from physical injury.[34]

When it comes to our health, when we start to see improvements, even in mental rehearsal, it reinforces belief in ourselves and where we are going. It puts you in control of your life, in your mind, and then in your reality.

According to research that looks at the brain during visualisation exercises, the neurons in our brains imagine our thoughts to be real-life actions.[35] Visualisation and action are intimately connected, and through imagining a movement, we mentally rehearse our intended physical movements. Our brains can learn over time to make our actions more automatic by creating and embedding new neural pathways – the paths of interconnected nerve cells that link what your body does to the brain impulses that control it.

There is also a body of research that shows that when we imagine ourselves feeling better or moving towards health, this happens, and that the opposite is also true.[38,39] Belief changes brain chemistry and brings physical changes – for better or worse.

Beliefs underpin the whole premise of 'the placebo effect', or more positively put, the 'perception effect'.[40] Rather than think of 'the placebo effect' as a form of trickery, conning you into feeling better, think of it instead as a mental retraining process that is the first step to getting to the health you want. Positive mental attitude is real when it comes to health habits.

You don't need to have a fantastic imagination to practise visualisation. The power of mental rehearsal is open to everyone. You may be someone who only hears words in your head, or sees colours or shadows when you close your eyes. It is okay – just begin to think about what you would like and how it looks, this in itself is a useful thing.

If you look at your life right now, how does it look? What do you feel happy and comfortable with, and where in your life would you like to see changes? Try answering these questions out loud or write your answers down.

It can be hard to see a bright future if we are ill or struggling. It is also easy to spend our time worrying about the bad things that *could* happen, imagining the worst outcomes rather than the best ones when we don't feel well. If we do this, we risk falling into a negative, depressive cycle and a defensive, familiar routine, not allowing the chance for new possibilities.

The moment that you wake up, what do you do first? Do you look at your phone? Start checking emails? Check Instagram, Facebook, Twitter, TikTok, news apps or WhatsApp? What do you do next? Get out of bed, clean your teeth, make breakfast, commute to work, chat to the same colleagues, work, eat lunch, come home, make dinner, get into bed . . .

In a very real sense, these habits become automatic, and direct you to the same tomorrow and future days based on what you have done on every past day.

How does this impact your body? It puts your emotional self and mental self into a similar repetitive process: you feel the same emotions each day, which lead to the same thoughts, which then lead you to make the same choices. *This is why it is crucial to make space for imagination and be open to change.* You don't have to perform a massive shake up to your basic routines, but simply by making space to imagine yourself and your life differently, you'll be open to the idea that you can do some of the things you have thought about.

A visualisation exercise

Set aside an hour to try this health habit. Write in the pages provided at the back of this book or turn to a fresh journal page. You need to be in a quiet, relaxing place – go somewhere you feel most comfortable. Ensure you will not be disturbed and have a good amount of time to concentrate.

What would you like to have, enjoy or work towards? (This can be something big, like combatting a health problem, or something small, like a walk every lunchtime.) Write everything down.

If you feel tempted to skip this bit, or unsure what you want to write, I urge you to instead grab a pen. Go do it now! Just make a start. Writing for even one minute will hopefully get some ideas flowing.

Help your body, mind and emotions relax as best they can by focusing on breathing slowly and steadily. Count to three slowly as you breathe in, and again as you breathe out.

How will you feel when you have achieved your goal? Imagine that emotion now, as best you can. Feel it.

You could say 'thank you' in your mind, with every out-breath, to reinforce the feeling of thankfulness.

Once you have got your breathing into a nice slow rhythm, start to visualise your future. Think about yourself in the first person and create an image of what you look like, paying close attention to the detail.

What can you see, hear, touch? Who is around you? Where are you? Engage your senses and make the environment as clear as you can. The more details you have, the more it will seem real.

Once you have a clear idea of how you look, focus on your emotions. Do you feel calm, happy, joyful, confident, proud? Can you imagine how that feels now?

Articulate what you are visualising and feeling. You could say: 'I am well', 'I am strong', 'I am pain-free', 'I am healthy', 'I am happy', 'I am walking', 'I am running', 'I am laughing'. These are just ideas; your personal choice may be different.

How do you feel? Return to your goal and visualise it as regularly as you can.

Think about what small changes you can make to your daily routine to help you get to that goal – have a look at the GLOVES framework for inspiration (page 280). Write your ideas down in your journal.

Hopefully you enjoyed that process.

Was it the first time you truly allowed your mind to wander, bringing you something new and unexpected?

Why not give yourself this time more often? Remember the science that shows repetition can change how we think for the better.

Reframing exercise

I love this tip from my friend and fellow GP, Dr Rangan Chatterjee, author of *Feel Better in Five*.[41] It comes from his 'reframe and release' exercise. Reframing your day sounds simple, but is a great way of boosting happiness and noticing the good in our lives. And it is a very straightforward thing to do. Simply write down three things that went well today. They could be small things like 'My mum called me', 'A car gave way for me at a junction', 'My dog was pleased to see me', 'The server at the shop smiled at me', or perhaps big things, if you had a particularly memorable day!

After you've written down each item in your journal, write what it means about the world. There is a lot of negativity in the news and on social media; outrage sells, after all. However, there are good, caring people everywhere. Sometimes reframing the day helps us remember this. A quick example: both my sons lost their backpacks while out and about on our last day on holiday in Berlin. They had their electronics and favourite souvenirs in their bags. We were soon flying back to London, but we decided to mentally retrace our steps and we called around all the places we had stopped to eat. One of the places we called miraculously had one of the bags! The person on the phone spoke English, and they promised to send the bag back to us in England. We could have chosen to focus on the negative event ruining our day and the bag that remained lost, or instead focus on the lessons learned about keeping our possessions safe, as well as focusing on all the other fun things we experienced on the trip and, of course, the cherry on top – the kindness of the server who was willing to send us the bag from another coun-try with all the items still inside. Our weekend in Berlin was all the richer for the way we chose to frame the events of that day. I know it might feel awkward at first, but it gets easier with practice, and is a powerful tool that will allow you to reframe your own emotions day to day and bring more posi-tivity to the days that come.

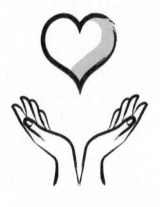

Love

What do I mean by love?

Love is a word some of us use a lot – from 'I just *love* pasta' to 'I love you' said to lovers, family, friends and children – while others never feel comfortable enough to say it out loud. Philosophers, theologians and now neuroscientists and clinicians think a lot about love.

For millennia, scholars have identified love as essential to human life, in its many forms. The Ancient Greek texts defined love in four ways: *eros* (romantic love), *philia* (love for friends and family), *storge* (a parent's love for their child) and *agape* (love for all mankind). *Agape* is also from the Christian tradition (the love of God towards his creation, and love mankind has for God, given without self-benefit).

In the Buddhist tradition, love similar to *agape* is defined as *karuna* (compassion, understanding and charity), *mudita* (joy), *maitri* (kindness) and *upeksha* (acceptance). The Hindu, Jain and Buddhist faiths also espouse the concept of *ahimsa* (the ethical principle of not causing harm to other living things). Hindu traditions talk of *atma prema* (a form of self-love cultivated by loving others), *bhakti* (a love that extends to all creation and God) and *maitri* (as in Buddhism, above).

The Shinto faith, meanwhile, has loving compassion at its core, with the figure of Quan Yin, the goddess of compassion, seen in statues throughout South East Asia.

Islamic scriptures state that without divine love there can be no human love.

In Judaism, and in the Torah, 'love your neighbour as yourself' is a central concept.

In Sikhism, *pyare* (love for God and creation), *sat* (truth), *santokh* (contentment), *daya* (compassion) and *nimrata* (humility) are the five virtues the gurus encourage Sikhs to aspire to.

Whatever you believe or don't believe, feelings of happiness, forgiveness, charity, joy and connection are biological processes.[1] Social conscience, family and community bonds are the foundation that society is built on. Choosing to love one another keeps life in order and gives us moral guidance to live by.

In this chapter, I want to talk about the health benefits of three different kinds of love.

1. Love for yourself/self-acceptance and self-kindness
2. Love for others
3. Love for your community

A gruelling exercise regime or a strict diet will, at some point, fail. This in part is due to the fact that these efforts were rooted more in exercising willpower, or as a result of negative self-talk, rather than being rooted in a genuine love for the 'self'. Positive self-regard allows us the opportunity to recognise we can do hard things, and maintain routines that will benefit us. It also allows for self-compassion when things don't go to plan.[4]

Why loving yourself keeps you healthy

Prioritising 'love' does not mean that you have to profess your undying love for everyone and everything in your life. I am sure there are many people and circumstances you can't honestly say that you love. Rather, it allows us to keep concepts like compassion, kindness and forgiveness not as distant ideals, but instead as values we live by each day.

Having 'loving thoughts' may seem to be an odd subject for a doctor to talk about, and although it is rarely expressed among my usual conversations about high-blood-pressure management and diabetes care, it is true to say that many of the patients I see feel a lack of love in their lives. I have come to observe that in *practical* terms, love can look like prioritising compassion, community and purpose.

I remember a patient of mine that we will call Sarah. She was struggling with her weight and mentioned to me that one of the ways she liked to relax was through food. She found comfort in evening snacking, and with young kids at home, she found it hard to make any time for herself, let alone for exercise. I'd known her for years and before she had her children, I knew she'd been a member of the local karate club. I asked her if she would ever consider getting back into it. She replied, 'I'm too fat now. And I just don't have the energy. I have forgotten so much of it, I'd just embarrass myself.' Sarah's comments were a reflection on her inner world – the things she says to herself every day. This wasn't just about not having time. This was about how she saw herself. We had a long chat and I asked her to think about what she would say to her sister if she was in Sarah's situation. She smiled and said, 'Hmm, I'd be a lot nicer to her than I am to myself, I know that . . .'.

I saw her a few months later and she happened to mention that she had decided to go back to her martial arts. She had found a fitness centre where she could take her toddler and train with other mums. She said she'd had a 'massive wake-up call' and wanted to be able to show her children that she had prioritised herself, and she wanted to show them that when they grow up, they could have a family and do things they enjoy too. Sarah was also going to an evening karate class, and so she found herself snacking less. She had made some new friends there as well as reconnecting with people she used to see at karate. She was even thinking of helping out at the kids' classes. Sarah had realised that the way she had been speaking to herself kept her stuck. When she had more compassion for herself, and decided to focus on what gave her a sense of purpose, she was able to feel part of her local community again too.

One of the big benefits of feeling connected to others is the sense of acceptance we feel when we are part of something bigger than ourselves. But it is important to feel accepted by ourselves too. If we don't feel this, it can be hard to persevere with friendships and community efforts. This also applies to lifestyle changes like the choices discussed in this book. With the smallest setback, many of us can withdraw, feeling overwhelmed or discouraged. Learning to accept the 'if they really knew me . . .' parts of ourselves is key to persevering with life changes, meeting new friends and deepening existing relationships.

Never lose compassion for yourself and the choices you have made up until this point. They are a part of your journey, and your story. Self-acceptance gives you the courage you need to grow, to heal, to find purpose, to love and to be loved. The practical tools I will give you in this section discussing values and forgiveness will all help you in the journey to accepting yourself just as you are.

In my surgery I see many people who define themselves by the opinions of parents, friends, employers, a spouse, an ex-spouse or even by past versions of themselves that do not serve who they are now, or who they want to be. This is completely natural, but it is also disempowering.

A lot of the ideas and concepts in this book are practical ways you can use to better understand who you are and what you need to feel good.

Your outside circumstances and responsibilities may not change straight away, and are not, in most cases, under your direct control. But the way you define yourself, and the practices you use to help you define yourself, are what can change. I'm talking about the idea of 'self-love', which might sound really strange coming from

a doctor. In this chapter I want to show you why it is important for
your health.

One of my patients came in to see me, and was struggling
with anxiety. We will call her Rebecca. She was a happily married
young professional working in accounting, and had an eight-
month-old daughter. She couldn't immediately see a reason why
her anxiety had escalated, so I asked her a bit about her day-to-day
routines. She could feel her anxiety rising.

We identified that anytime she had to leave her baby or plan
for her return to work, she would feel a sense of panic. She noticed
racing thoughts around her daughter's safety and her ability to be
able to return to work. I asked her to tell me what those thoughts
were. She broke down in tears: 'You're not good enough, you can't
even stop your baby from crying, you're useless, you're stupid,
you're pathetic, you'll be rubbish at your job when you go back,
you can't even remember anything now, you'll never remember all
the things you need to be good at your job . . .' – and so the list
went on. A barrage of abuse.

I asked her how she'd feel if a friend had said these things to
her. She looked at me wryly and admitted she probably wouldn't
be their friend anymore. I asked her about the first time she had
had thoughts like this, and she recalled that her father had often
spoken to her negatively as a child. He'd say, 'You're ugly, you're
stupid, you're so lazy' on a regular basis, and she described him as
a highly critical influence in her life.

A career in accounting was one of the ways in which Rebecca
had sought his approval, as he himself was an accountant. Her
self-talk had been shaped by the words she had internalised from
her father. Most of us don't need such an obvious source of criticism to become self-critical, but for her it was a pattern which had
started very young.

I asked Rebecca to imagine what she might say to her own

daughter to soothe her from anxiety. Reframing her own response to anxiety helped. I asked her to imagine someone in her life that she would describe as the 'perfect nurturer'. Rebecca chose her aunt. I asked Rebecca to imagine what her aunt might say to her. As we talked through her ideas, I could see her expression shifting and her physiology calming. She even began to smile when she imagined her aunt saying, 'You've already achieved so much. I am so proud of you. Your daughter is thriving. You were competent at your job before you left and you'll get back into it just as quickly. You have so much support and love, and you have always been conscientious and strived to be the best that you can.'

I asked Rebecca to write these ideas down and keep them to hand to refer back to. (See page 73 for the 'good guide' exercise.)

We also found a breathing technique that Rebecca found calming, that she could easily do whenever she felt her body or thoughts shifting towards panic.

I want you to talk to yourself

Have you ever noticed how it makes you feel when a family member or a work colleague speaks harshly to you? Very often we will internalise the negative comments they make, and these will affect how we view ourselves and the world. This is especially true in our childhood, a stage of development where our perception is often that the course of our lives is controlled primarily by our own thoughts and actions, more than by external circumstances. According to psychologist Jean Piaget, early childhood is a time when our so-called 'locus of control' is skewed towards things being 'because of us'. We are wired to take everything personally.[3] Harsh criticism or neglect during this time in our lives can result in a number of thinking patterns, including self-criticism ('I'm useless'), black and white thinking ('I *always* get things wrong'), poor boundaries (agreeing to things we don't want), learned helplessness ('I can't do anything about it') and chronic self-blame ('It's all my fault'). Remember, recognising patterns of thinking does not mean we blame our caregivers. Our parents, for the most part, do the very best they can with the tools they were given. (It is also possible that these thinking patterns have other origins.)

A work colleague once spoke very critically towards me back when I was a junior doctor, and I asked him, 'Why did you give me this feedback in such a negative way?' He responded: 'If you think that was harsh, try living inside my head. I am far harsher to myself than I'd ever be to anyone else, including you.'

Our inner world shapes our outer world, and our responses to the people around us. Many of us go through life without looking at how our own patterns of thought and behaviour contribute to patterns of experience – at home and at work. It is important to be aware of the parts of ourselves we feel proud of, but also the parts of ourselves we may not like as much, or that we want to change. Jungian psychology teaches us that the things we find most aggravating in other people, and our reactions to their behaviour, can reveal deep-seated fears and unresolved issues within ourselves. In other words: what irritates you about someone else is likely to be something that also irritates you about yourself.

Although this concept is somewhat jarring, it is also a golden opportunity to learn more about ourselves. Strong emotional reactions can also happen when we unconsciously attribute our own thoughts, feelings, and behaviours to other people – often as a way of avoiding or denying them in ourselves.[3] For example, if we have a tendency to be critical of others, we can become easily irritated by someone that we perceive as being critical of us. As Carl Jung said, 'Until you make the unconscious conscious, it will direct your life and you will call it fate.' The purpose of introducing this concept here is to help you create more awareness in your life. If we can recognise the so-called 'shadow' parts of ourselves, in Jung's words, it's easier for us to feel accepting of ourselves as we are, and subsequently more accepting of other people. Acceptance is a form of self-compassion. And self-compassion is a form of love.

Positive self-talk exercise

What does your self-talk sound like? What type of things do you criticise yourself for? Your appearance? Your abilities? Perhaps your personality, or your likeability when you compare yourself to others? I want you to write down some of the more negative things you say to yourself. Be really honest. Imagine that the person saying all those things in your head is now standing in front of you. What would they look like? What is the expression on their face when they say these things, and what tone of voice are they using? How do you feel having them stood right in front of you? What do you think their intentions towards you are?

Your self-talk is the person you have to live with every day for the rest of your life. You need to live with an honest friend, rather than an adversary always on the attack. It will take practice and repetition to build up those neural networks that wire you for self-compassion. Notice when the self-critic pops up (which may be quite a lot at first), and talk to the critic with kindness.

Now I want you to imagine what a compassionate person would say to you – a person who is honest and kind, someone who is supportive and wants the best for you. Can you remember a time when someone in your life has been compassionate towards you? How did they look at you and what kinds of things did they say?

When the inner critic takes over, don't try to block them – they will shout louder. It is okay to have negative thoughts. Thoughts are not facts about yourself, and they come and go. Accept the thoughts and feelings are there. Then consider what a good friend or mentor would say to you in reply. Not empty platitudes, but words of encouragement, accountability and honesty.

Positive role modelling

The concept of a 'perfect nurturer' comes from compassion-focused therapy (CFT), which is a type of psychotherapy that centres on the emotions behind people's thoughts. By way of comparison, cognitive behavioural therapy (CBT) focuses on thought patterns and behaviour change. The idea with CFT is that mental and emotional healing can occur when we can foster compassionate feelings towards ourselves and others. Although it is less well known as a concept, a recent systematic review has shown that it is an effective tool in helping people with mental health struggles.[2]

Who inspires you?

Making changes in life is so much easier when we have people around us who are doing the same thing. We are all inspired in one way or another by those who have come before us, or who have helped us to dream and imagine a different version of ourselves. We have to hold these dreams gently, and give thanks to those who inspired them – even if they have died or are people we are never likely to meet.

I am so lucky to have had countless mentors. My mother taught me the power of unconditional love. My sister taught me the emotional comfort of honesty and connection. My husband has provided steadfast wisdom, insights and affection, and has opened my eyes to the practicalities of plant-based nutrition for performance. My eldest son has taught me so much about integrity, kindness and creativity, and I love seeing the world through his eyes. My youngest son reminds me to be grateful above all else for moments of love, joy and laughter. Further afield, I have admired many physicians, psychologists, musicians, teachers and friends who show me what living with vision and values can achieve. There are people in that journey whom I have admired from afar, and others I've known for a lifetime. The mentors we can call upon in our own lives are arguably the most powerful. Think whether there is someone you know who embodies values you admire. Could you arrange to spend more time with them? Are there any mentors in your own life? Either in your social circle or online?

The good guide exercise

Who might your 'perfect nurturer' be? If you can't think of anyone in your life, is there a character from a TV show, a film or online who you could imagine being a good mentor? You can choose more than one person. Write about them in your journal.

Now, if there are negative thoughts you are struggling with about yourself, what would that person say? What practical advice might they give?

Having a coach, guide or mentor to whom you can talk — and share whatever challenge you are currently facing, how you feel about it and what you ultimately want — is priceless. Think of this person — real or imaginary. What do you think this 'perfect nurturer' might say to you? Imagine the words in detail. Write them down if it helps. It usually does! Then move forward with your day.

Journalling can be an incredibly helpful tool, and is surprisingly effective in promoting greater awareness of self and creating shifts in mindset, allowing you to express yourself openly and to reflect on previous entries with greater objectivity.

Love letter-writing exercise

Now it's time to write some things down. Focus on the kind words that people have said to you in the past. Use this as inspiration to write a letter.

If you can't write to yourself, can you imagine a best friend who is struggling and doing their best to change? What would you say to them? How would you help them? Write this down in a letter to yourself. Don't worry; nobody else has to read it. It is simply a way to train your mind towards more self-acceptance. Research shows that compassionate self-talk helps us to fear failure less, and try again more willingly when we do fail.

Positive statements

'Sticks and stones may break my bones, but words will never hurt me.' I used to say that to the kids who would call me names when I was at school. But the truth is, words can hurt us a great deal. We've all been hurt by words. And for many of us, as we grow into adults, the words we say to *ourselves* are often far harsher than we would ever say to other people, as you have seen in the stories shared earlier. This is where interrupting negative thought patterns and self-talk can be so powerful. There's real value in patting ourselves on the back from time to time, accepting compliments from others graciously and noticing the good stuff about ourselves.

Have you heard of affirmations? Affirmations are positive statements that can help change your outlook on the world when you say them to yourself regularly, or write them down in a journal. Ancient Hindu and Buddhism traditions have used mantra-based meditations to focus on universal truths for thousands of years. More recently, seventeenth-century philosopher René Descartes (who coined the phrase 'I think, therefore I am'; *'Cogito, ergo sum'*) was thought to use affirmations and, pressing fast forward to the 1930s, Napoleon Hill's book *Think and Grow Rich* was the first of its kind to use positive affirmations to improve chances of success in various aspects of life.[5]

Studies support the idea that the words we choose matter.[6] Research also shows that positive words can activate the reward system in the brain, which can have an impact on the way we experience both emotional and physical pain.[7,8] Affirmations are a completely free and easy way to improve your day, if you are in the headspace to enjoy them.

An important note: some positive affirmations *do not* help people with low self-esteem, especially if they feel untrue. I think the important thing here is to repeat positive statements *only* if they feel true to you. If they feel wrong, or you notice that your mind immediately rejects them, find alternative statements that align with where you currently are instead. For example, if 'I am beautiful' doesn't feel comfortable to you, perhaps 'My body is strong and I accept my flaws' feels more true and easier to say with conviction. Or, if you are prone to binge eating, rather than saying 'I eat healthy foods' or even 'I want to eat healthy foods', you could say, 'I want to feel empowered to eat healthy foods'.

Bottom line – if affirmations don't make you feel good, try something else.

I have included a list of affirmation suggestions to inspire you to find your own.

You could say one of them out loud to start your day, or whisper it to yourself before you sleep. Repetition is also helpful – try saying the phrase five times in a way that feels authentic to you.

If this feels awkward, writing the words down five times for yourself in your journal can be a good place to start.

Affirmations

1. I am in the right place, at the right time, for me.
2. I am loved for who I am.
3. My mind and body are strong and resilient.
4. I listen to my body and take things at my own pace.
5. I trust my body – it knows what it's doing.
6. My self-care is important and worth making time for.
7. I give myself permission to rest.
8. I can let my true self be seen by others.
9. I deserve to nourish my body.

10. I move my body to look after myself.
11. I love moving my body in ways that I enjoy.
12. I make space for the unexpected.
13. I am good enough.
14. I am as kind and loving to myself as I am to others.
15. I am deliberate in the choices I make.
16. I am enough.
17. I am listening to my inner voice.
18. I am thankful for the positive things in my life.
19. I treat my body with respect and compassion.
20. My history does not define me.
21. I am patient and kind to myself every day.
22. I am grateful. Thank you.
23. Change is a natural part of life.
24. I speak to myself as I would to a close friend.
25. My life is what I make of it.
26. My thoughts are unique and they can make a difference to the world.
27. I accept every part of me. Even the messy parts.
28. I am willing to let go of my expectations.
29. I look for ways to support those around me, without expectation of them reciprocating.
30. I remember the things that are important to me.

Inspire, don't compare

If you follow accounts on social media that inspire you or make you feel connected, great.

If your scrolling finds you comparing yourself to others, feeling that your life isn't good enough, or your body isn't good enough, then you are actively damaging your self-esteem with every scroll.

Can you pay attention as you scroll to identify if certain posts cause you to feel negatively about yourself? Is there content in your feed that you don't want to focus on? Unfollow, block or hide these pages.

We tend to have fairly simple and singular ways of comparing ourselves to others – I wish I had their career, their legs, their skin, their hair, their muscles. But ask yourself: would you want to really swap your life with theirs? Would you want their family dynamic, their mental health, their history, their relationship with alcohol, food, work? Maybe not. Filters and highlights make it harder to see the negatives in other's lives, but they are always there, because that is life!

Are there aspects of your life you would never want to lose? Write them down and treasure them.

Start accepting compliments

Has someone said something nice about you that your mind immediately rejected? Do you instinctively find excuses as to why their compliment is not genuine, or undeserved? People with low self-esteem can have a hard time accepting positive feedback. Work on noticing how you respond to a compliment; if you tend to reject it, you will not only reinforce negative beliefs about yourself, but you can also (unintentionally) make others feel rejected when their kind words are dismissed.

Next time someone pays you a compliment, say 'thank you'. Write the compliment down later. Collecting positive data points helps to crowd out that tendency that many of us have to notice the negative. It will also help you genuinely notice the good stuff in other people, and feel freer to share a compliment with them.

Practise self-acceptance

Do the words 'I love myself' make you cringe? Don't worry, you're not alone! But it is true that finding a way to accept things about ourselves that are less than perfect will help us to accept the imperfections in other people more easily. Do you have regrets? Most of us do. However, shame is not a good motivator. When people feel shame (i.e. 'I am a bad person') they also feel worthless and exposed. Rather than motivating reparative action (like guilt might; 'I did a bad thing'), the painful shame experience can instead cause a defensive response. When shamed, people want to escape, hide, deny responsibility and blame others.[9] A more helpful emotion, whether following guilt, or simply when reflecting on ourselves, is self-acceptance.

Self-acceptance does not mean that we 'let ourselves get away with' unhealthy behaviour. Nor does it mean saying and doing whatever we want, regardless of whether it hurts others, so we can 'stay true to ourselves'. We don't want to continue making poor decisions.

But when we aim to accept who we are, in spite of regrets, it can help us to make decisions that we can feel proud of in the future. How can we start to do this?

Actively seek to do things that make you feel proud of yourself. If you value kindness, aim to do something kind every day. Do you value curiosity? Aim to learn something new every day. If you value joy, do something to make your friends, family, colleagues smile today.

When you take positivity-boosting actions intentionally, it can begin the process of reprogramming your mind to feel more positive about yourself too.

The importance of positive relationships

Research suggests that our self-esteem is largely influenced by people within our social circles.[10] This starts with our parents, and as we get older, our peers and friendships often reflect our values and interests. But these relationships can also reflect – and affect – our self-esteem. Spend time with the people who make you feel respected, valued and cared for. Show the people you love or admire that you notice the good stuff about them, if it feels natural to do so.

We are social creatures who are hardwired for connection. It is embedded in our biology. Ironically, in a time when we are more digitally connected than ever, there is a sharp increase in the number of people experiencing loneliness, social isolation and depression.[11]

Several large studies point to loneliness and isolation as risk factors in premature death.[12-15] When we feel we have been rejected socially, the amygdala – the region of the brain associated with threat – activates in the same way as it would against a physical threat, going into overdrive.[16] The resulting anxiety can compromise the immune system and affect long-term physical health.[17]

Similar mechanisms play a role in many diseases, such as diabetes and cancer. This is not just an issue for older people; according to the UK government's 'Tackling Loneliness' strategy review, reported loneliness is higher for people who are 16 to 24 years old, female, renting, single or widowed, living with a mental health condition, have lower neighbourhood belonging and for those with lower local social trust.[13] This shows that the importance of meaningful emotional connection is something that spans all ages.

It is worth noting that social isolation and loneliness do not necessarily go together. Some people may be alone and not feel lonely, whereas some people may be surrounded by others, yet not feel emotionally connected to them and feel great loneliness. Studies highlight that many who reported feeling lonely were married, lived with others and were not clinically depressed.[18] If your relationships don't make you feel safe and accepted, it can impact your health in the same negative ways as loneliness can. Giving time to these intimate relationships and friendships is an important way to prevent loneliness over the course of time.

The healing power of belonging

Why is it that a sense of belonging can be so healing for us? From what I see in my interactions with patients, belonging is created through the power of feeling listened to and feeling understood. Conversely, truly listening to other people, and trying to understand their point of view, can be the most healing of gifts we can give to a person. It's amazing how many patients I see who say 'I feel so much better now', when all that had changed was that they'd had the chance to express their fears to someone who listened intently.

From birth, a loving caregiver (usually a parent) gives us love, time and support. It is free, and unlike shiny new toys and fancy holidays, love is the one thing the brains of human babies seem to need more than anything else. The love of a caregiver has actually been shown to help cushion us from the blows of heartbreak, adolescent angst and even exam and career stress years later.[19] Studies on epigenetics show that the first year of life is crucial to the early wiring and pruning of the 700 to 1,000 synaptic connections per second that are made during this incredible period of brain growth.[19] It is the ongoing loving interactions and communication with a baby that can lead to the creation of brain pathways that help us make memories, form relationships and allow for learning and logic to develop.[20]

Our parents provide the blueprint from which our understanding of love and connection grows. Some of us are not lucky enough to have at least one parent who showed us love in a way that we could feel accepted and safe. But if you didn't have that experience, you can learn to love at any age.[21] Trust that these wounds can be healed, and even if we feel we are not, the truth is we are *all* healers – of ourselves and of each other. That is why belonging can be so powerful. We can help people heal in small ways: through touch, through forgiveness, through listening, through an unexpected kindness or simply through the grace of allowing someone to be, just as they are. If you are reading this, and you feel that you did not experience the love of at least one caregiver in your early years, I'd strongly recommend seeking the help of a therapist if you can. I'd also suggest journalling, in order to sort through some of the feelings and patterns this brings up in your life. How might it have affected your thoughts, and your perceptions of the people around you? Did you have a pattern of pushing people away before they could reject you? Do you seek out relationships that, in hindsight, did not feel safe or healthy? Knowing how these patterns come up in your life is an empowering thing to understand. Finding compassion for yourself will also help you find compassion for your absent caregiver, and perhaps a realisation that whoever was born into that scenario would have faced the same circumstances that you did. It was never because of you.

For some people, a strong sense of belonging comes from being around those who share their beliefs and cultural values. For others, it's shared hobbies and passions, or being with people that share the same priorities, goals and life stages.[20] Strong links with others who live in a community with you are one of the key protective factors against loneliness and poor health in our old age, even for those who had to deal with childhood adversity.[21]

When you feel isolated or lonely, it can be hard to take steps to feel a sense of belonging. Here are a handful of simple ideas allowing you to be intentional when it comes to fostering new connections:

- **Focus on others.** If you have enough energy after family commitments, volunteering can be hugely rewarding and is scientifically proven to benefit physical and mental wellbeing, and reduce stress and anxiety.[22] As well as helping you to develop stronger social networks, it can help improve life skills and even employability, if this is something that is important to you. There are many organisations within communities that are actively looking for people to help them.

- **Remember the saying 'If you want a friend, be a friend.'** Don't wait for someone else to make the first move! Text, call or email the people you like, proactively arrange to meet up and show them you care about the things that are going on for them.

- **Make time for your passions.** If you join a group that has a shared interest, you will have at least one thing in common with everyone there. It can be anything. What are you into? There will be a group of like-minded people out there for you.

- **Support a friend.** Do you have friends who are part of something that interests you? A good friend of mine convinced me to accompany her to a local kickboxing class to help motivate her. I would never have chosen it, but I ended up reaching a blue belt in kickboxing and kept attending classes long after she had stopped going. You never know what or who could inspire you to experience a different version of yourself. I certainly never imagined myself performing a jab-cross-hook combination and then leaping into the air for a flying kick . . .

❈ **Start online but take it offline.** The internet has made making new connections easier than ever. You can find special-interest groups for everything you can imagine, and Google is the answer to finding groups within your local area. However, if you never make it from behind your computer screen or phone, then you will find it hard to reap the rewards of any connection you make. Sites like meetup.com are a great way to find a real community near where you live or work.

❈ **Laugh!** This is perhaps an unusual tip from a doctor. One of my favourite things to do to invite love into each day is smiling and laughing. Smiling is a way of connecting to others, as well as boosting your own mood by stimulating the parasympathetic nervous system, which releases pain-controlling endorphins and enhances positive emotions.[23] Even watching a funny film can have physiological effects to improve blood flow and blood vessel flexibility.[24] But laughter not only helps you, it is also powerfully contagious and can strengthen your social bonds and sense of shared connection more than almost anything else. We have an instinct for facial mimicry – and this neurological network also has the power to improve our sense of empathy.[25] Facial researchers even found, in one study, that smiling makes you more attractive to others.[26]

A happier workplace

Before retirement, we spend most of our time at work when we are not sleeping. So this is an important part of life to consider when looking at how we can bring positive interactions into our day-to-day routines. Does your job make you happy? Do you look forward to your work, or feel it gives you a sense of self-worth? Do you feel accepted and supported by colleagues?

Tips for a happier workplace

- ✸ **Can you make a valued friend at work?** Having a friend to share the day with makes work more enjoyable, satisfying and potentially more productive. Can you invite a trusted work colleague out for coffee, tea, lunch, drinks or dinner?

- ✸ **Do you enjoy your work?** Can you plan to move jobs? Many people get stuck with a job they no longer enjoy and don't think they can leave. You have options. Research shows relying on listening to what your parents or your peers think you should do, or choosing a job for more prestige or a bigger pay cheque will not be the ultimate answer to happiness at work.[20] Make the most of your holidays. Too many people don't use all their accrued holiday time. It is so important to your health that you take time away from work. Use your holiday leave and plan for adventures to enrich your life, and you can share them with your work colleagues when you get back!

- ✸ **Unplug.** Do you always really need to check emails and messages outside of the working day or is this an unhealthy habit? If this is expected of you, could you start putting boundaries in place, or set up an out-of-office notification to use at the end of your working day?

❀ **Can you bike or walk to work?** If you have a commute of an hour or more in your car or on public transport, can you get out for a walk in your working day? (More on the importance of going outside from page 103.)

❀ **Goals are not just to hit your work targets and be seen as successful.** They should also include targets to ensure that you love what you do, find your work meaningful and feel a sense of purpose from it. (See also visualisation on page 56.)

Has this section sparked any ideas in you? If so, take a moment to write them in the notes section at the back of this book, or in your journal.

How does forgiveness affect health?

I had a patient, let's call her Sara, who confided to me that she had never managed to forgive her husband for having relationships with other women. He had done this several times, and when describing this to me, she had simply said: 'I turned a blind eye. I knew it was happening, but what could I do? What would people say? How could I go on alone?'

She grew up in a time and place where arranged marriages were common, and she wondered if this was why he felt the need to be with other women. Perhaps he had never really loved her? She knew he had not chosen her – his parents had. She had been the dutiful wife, looking after the family and protecting their kids from the truth of their father's habits. But she resented him.

The emotional effects of this private warfare took its toll on her body. She had been coming to see me with chronic pain issues and fatigue for a very long time. Each time she came, we discussed her life and state of mind. She would shrug a lot, glance at me sadly, then stare into the distance, saying she could not change anything and life was just as it was 'meant to be'. But she kept returning with all-over body pain, fibromyalgia and headaches.

Sara had also developed breast cancer and was undergoing a rigorous course of treatment for this. Her cancer had taken over their married life and meant many trips to the hospital. As I saw her for a follow-up during her treatment, something strange happened. Her aches and pains had begun to diminish. Despite her rigorous chemotherapy schedule and worsening prognosis, her headaches disappeared, and she came in to see me with a smile.

She said, 'I am feeling much better, thank you, Doctor.'

It turned out that Sara's husband would take her for the hospital trips she needed for her cancer therapy and would sit with her, hold her hand and make her cups of tea. He had told her how much he loved her, how he would not know what to do if she left him.

'How did this feel?' I asked her.

'Like I am truly loved,' she said. 'After all this time, I matter to him. I see this now.'

'Have you talked about your feelings?' I asked.

'No need. I forgive him. He loved me all along. And now I know it. I feel it. And that is all I need to know.'

I loved talking to Sara about her journey to forgiveness. This is her story, and she found emotional comfort in a way that did not involve discussing her past. Generally, I'd advise that it is crucial to be able to talk about your feelings when you have been betrayed in a relationship. If the relationship is to continue, important changes in how you relate to each other and express your needs and boundaries are vital. In Sara's case, forgiveness came from within. Trying to forgive, and seeking love: these are gifts we give to ourselves.

Whether it is a recent row with your partner or a long-term resentment of a member of your family, unresolved conflict can affect our health in many ways.[27] Anger and hurt can cause numerous physical changes in our bodies. Studies consistently show that the act of forgiving someone can reduce pain and blood pressure, improve cholesterol levels, improve immune function, and lower the risk of anxiety and depression.[28] As we get older, research also shows there is a closer connection between forgiveness and health, so the older you are, the more physical benefits there are to offering forgiveness.[29]

In my experience, patients with chronic pain are commonly misunderstood. They are treated unfairly, and can find themselves excluded from many parts of normal social, family and work life. This can leave people with feelings of anger, resentment and hopelessness. Data shows that active training in forgiveness can actually reduce pain perception for people who are suffering with chronic disease conditions.[30] We are often told that forgiveness is not for the person who has wronged you, but really for the person who has chosen to forgive. To see this wise principle improving a chronic illness is hugely exciting.

We cannot change the past. We cannot change the situation or the person whom we feel wronged by. But we can control the effect these events have on our body, mind and spirit moving forward. We can change the physiological effect of that event by changing our mind about what it means.[31] So, in this sense, we have the potential to be able to change the past. For example, if we feel our parents did not love us the way we feel we deserved, or they made mistakes, it is easy to get caught in emotional quicksand, to get trapped by hurt from the past.

Think about the circumstances and limitations they faced in

their life that have impacted them and shaped how they respond to the world around them. They will have had their own struggles, pains, and sorrow. Can you see things from a different perspective?

To forgive does not mean we have to accept or condone what they have done, or justify their behaviour. We don't have to even keep them as a part of our lives. It simply means not holding that hurt, that wrong, close to you anymore. Looking forward rather than reliving the past. Letting the emotion go. It is a choice we may have to make more than once when we feel let down or disappointed by someone. However, striving to forgive can boost our self-esteem and give us a sense of inner strength.[32] A nice gift to ourselves.

Have you hurt someone in your life? Have you done something that you wish you really hadn't? Join the club. Admitting you were wrong takes courage. Apologising without excuses takes vulnerability. It can be the hardest thing to do. But doing so, wholeheartedly, will set you free from regret, from pain and from shame. You will feel better.

Forgiveness letter exercise

One effective way I have seen people forgive is by using their imaginations to let go of resentment and anger. You may be wondering, does this work if you don't forgive them just yet? Would saying the words disingenuously be more harmful to the process? No. Remember, this is an exercise for you, not for them. Saying the words to yourself with intention, even if they're not yet true, can be helpful in getting you that bit closer to feeling peace. And peace in your own heart is a gift you give to yourself.

- ❀ Write down on a piece of paper the person who has hurt you and the reasons why.
- ❀ Next, close your eyes and visualise the person. Have a conversation with them, in which you tell them exactly what they have done, how it has made you feel and what you would like from them.
- ❀ Once you have said everything you want, imagine telling them you are going to do your best to forgive them. At the end of the conversation, tell them: 'I forgive you'.
- ❀ On the piece of paper, next to your notes, write: 'I forgive you'.
- ❀ If you need to repeat the exercise over a number of days, do so, until you feel lighter. One day you may find that the feelings have simply melted away.

This is similar to the meaning-maker exercise (on page 37) that helps us to view hurt in a different way. It is a reframing of your experience, to allow you more of an opportunity to let go of the negative emotions attached to it.

Loving-kindness exercise

This is a well-known practice derived from a loving-kindness meditation, also known as 'metta meditation' (in Pali, the language in which ancient Buddhist scripts are written), and it refers to a mental state of unselfish and unconditional kindness to all beings. The word *mettā* means directing goodwill and love towards everyone. It helps us to feel increased compassion and kindness and, importantly, it helps us to forgive others. Don't be put off by the idea of meditation if you have struggled with it in the past. Think of this instead as a time out for yourself, where you make time to deal with things holding you back that you might not normally give time to.

- ❀ Sit in a comfortable position with your back straight and your hands on your knees or in your lap. Close your eyes and breathe gently.
- ❀ Focus on your breath as you breathe in and out and try to quieten your mind.
- ❀ Imagine yourself at peace, with perfect inner calmness and wellness. Focus on breathing out tension and breathing in love.
- ❀ If your attention drifts, bring it slowly back to the exercise.
- ❀ Once you are calm, picture the person you would like to forgive and send them love and happiness. Say in your mind: 'May you be happy, may you be safe, may you be loved.' Notice how you feel. Tell them you are ready to forgive them, and let go.
- ❀ When you feel the meditation is complete, gently open your eyes.

Important note: If you have experienced an abusive situation, this forgiveness exercise alone may not be appropriate for you, and I recommend you also seek help from a therapist.

We all need a reason to live

Do you have a sense of purpose? It can be a tough question to answer. For some this concept can seem quite daunting, especially in our teenage years. Or at a time of life when we might feel trapped into a certain path we chose years ago, or a way of being that no longer serves us.

The Japanese concept of *ikigai* combines the terms *iki*, meaning 'alive' or 'life', and *gai*, meaning 'benefit' or 'worth'. It's similar to the French term *raison d'etre*, or 'reason for being'. Both are about living a life of meaning. *Ikigai* originated from Japanese medical traditions that recognised our physical wellbeing is affected by our emotions and by having a sense of purpose in our lives. Neuroscientist Ken Mogi says that *ikigai* is an ancient and familiar concept for the Japanese, and can be poetically described as 'waking up to joy'. It also relates to the concept of flow, a state of being which happens when you are in your 'zone', a sweet spot where we apply ourselves with effort to something, e.g. art or an athletic achievement. It is important to note that *ikigai* does not refer only to our *personal* fulfillment, but also encompasses others and society as a whole. The premise is that you find something that you are passionate about, and then figure out a medium through which to express that passion, ideally where you can earn an income too. This is a marvellous idea, but it can also put a lot of pressure on our psyche if we haven't found that one thing we want to do, or a way of making money that has meaning for us.

Ikigai hints at the idea that we are all born for some higher purpose, but the reality is that for a lot of us, it's enough to be able to afford to put food on the table for our families, or be able to deal with a debilitating disease each day, and find time for our family. With this in mind, I'd like to share a parable written by an Italian psychiatrist Roberto Assagioli.[32] Three stonecutters from the fourteenth century were interviewed about their job building a cathedral. When the first stonecutter was asked what he was doing, the man replied bitterly that he was cutting stones into blocks. He had cut stones into blocks over and over again, and would continue to do so until he died. The second stonecutter was also cutting stones into blocks, but he saw his task differently. With warmth, he said that he was earning a living for his family, so that his children had clothes and food, and his family a home that they fill with love. But it was the third stonecutter who truly channelled his *ikigai*. In a joyous voice, he described the thrill he felt in being a part of building this great cathedral, so strong and mighty that it will stand as a lighthouse of wonder and prayer for a thousand years, for many generations of people he will never know. A legacy to the divine. All three men were doing exactly the same thing with competence and skill. But finding meaning in a familiar task brings it a layer of joy, gratitude and purpose that was otherwise hidden from view.

Psychologists have consistently found that people with a clear sense of purpose in life tend to have better brain and mental health function.[33] One study of 6,800 teachers in China showed a link between a sense of purpose, resilience and stress. Those with a greater sense of purpose were better able to manage stressful events.[34] For younger people, research shows that teenagers and young adults who lead a more purposeful life reported higher self-esteem, less delinquency and better wellbeing.[35] Having a sense of purpose as we age also imparts important health benefits. It can reduce the risk of heart disease, strokes and dementia.[36-38]

So, what does this mean and how do we find purpose?

I had a patient a few years ago who was training to be a funeral director. It was all he'd ever wanted to do. This idea as a vocation may surprise many of you, especially as we live in a society that likes to keep death private, often hidden from sight and conversation. He described to me the great sense of purpose he found in preparing the body of the person who had died, for them to look their best as their grieving families come to say their last goodbyes. He enjoyed guiding people through their hardest of times, knowing he could make the loss of a loved one a little bit easier to bear for the families that are left behind.

This resonated with me on many levels. In my training, many of the medical students that trained alongside me vowed never to be GPs. They saw it as a path of boredom, dealing with constant coughs and colds. I saw things differently. Having a window into the lives and stories of thousands of people over their whole lifetimes is a true gift. Having a person willing to share with me their vulnerabilities, fears and pain is a tremendous honour and is something I cherish and feel honoured to be a part of. That is how I see my work.

Practical ways to feel a sense of purpose

Purpose does not have to be a grand gesture or change-the-world achievement. All you need to do is ask yourself two simple questions. Take a moment to think:

- ❀ What is important to me?
- ❀ What could I do *today* to serve what is most important to me?

Tom Rath once said, 'You cannot become anything you want, but you can become everything you are.' If we take the time to ask ourselves these two simple questions, we begin to build up a personal picture of the puzzle pieces needed to have purpose in our own lives. These questions can take us in subtle directions that we would not have expected. Purpose can then emerge from these little habits that we slot into our daily lives. Allow yourself the time to pause. To question whether the path you are taking is the one that makes you feel satisfied. Noticing where your passions truly lie is an interesting exercise. Sometimes, we find that what brings us joy is not always the thing we expected. These unexpected insights help us to build a life that energises us.

An exercise to find your values

A really simple way to hone your sense of purpose each day is to say the three values that are most important to you before you start your day. You could think carefully and choose the three values that you would like to drive you in life.

Think about what you want your efforts to represent. What kind of person you hope to be.

Remember, values are not the same as goals. For example, if your value is 'compassion', your goal might be to visit a relative, or to pop some items in the food bank drop-off on your next supermarket shopping trip. If your value is 'health', your goal might be to move your body (even for five minutes) each day, or to try a breathing exercise.

Sometimes it helps to think of the reason behind your value. So if you think of your value as 'money', ask yourself why. If it is so you can afford to feed your family, and you grew up living in a low-income household, your value might actually be 'security'. If you chose money because you want to be able to jump on a plane at the drop of a hat, or say yes to doing things that excite you, then your underlying value is likely to be 'freedom'.

Here's a list of values, to get your imagination going:

Abundance	Contribution	Human Rights
Acceptance	Creativity	Humility
Accountability	Credibility	Humour
Achievement	Curiosity	Inclusiveness
Adventure	Daring	Independence
Advocacy	Decisiveness	Individuality
Altruism	Dedication	Innovation
Ambition	Dependability	Inspiration
Appreciation	Diversity	Intelligence
Attractiveness	Empathy	Intuition
Autonomy	Encouragement	Joy
Balance	Engagement	Justice
Being the best	Enthusiasm	Kindness
Being proactive	Ethics	Knowledge
Benevolence	Excellence	Leadership
Boldness	Expressiveness	Learning
Brilliance	Fairness	Love
Calmness	Family	Loyalty
Caring	Friendships	Open-mindedness
Challenge	Flexibility	Optimism
Charity	Freedom	Originality
Cheerfulness	Fun	Passion
Cleverness	Generosity	Peace
Collaboration	Grace	Perfection
Commitment	Gratitude	Performance
Communication	Greed	Personal
Community	Growth	development
Compassion	Happiness	Philanthropy
Consistency	Health	Playfulness
Cooperation	Honesty	Popularity

Power	Security	Transparency
Preparedness	Self-Interest	Trust
Professionalism	Service	Unity
Recognition	Social Connection	Variety
Reliability	Spirituality	Warmth
Respect	Stability	Wealth
Risk-taking	Thoughtfulness	Wisdom
Romance	Tolerance	Wit
Safety	Traditions	

What are your values? Jot them down below. For each one, ask yourself: why is this value important to you? How has it shaped your life?

Value 1:

Value 2:

Value 3:

Once you have chosen your three values, repeat them while looking at yourself in the mirror as you clean your teeth. A 'values check-in' is helpful as a way of figuring out if your day-to-day habits match the values you hold as important.

I promise you – it will change how you feel about yourself, how you perform and the outcomes you experience. One study, undertaken by German researchers in 2015, demonstrates just how critical it is to know our values, especially when faced with stress.[39] Study participants had to undergo an objectively stressful experience. They were told they had just five minutes to prepare a presentation in front of a panel of judges, who had been secretly instructed to give no positive reactions. The participants were given a pen and paper to prepare, and then they had to sit in front of the panel, with a video camera and audio recording equipment. Then their paper was unexpectedly taken away. If they stopped their presentation, they were told to continue, until they had been speaking for at least five minutes. Once they had done their presentation, they had to do a mental arithmetic challenge. If they made a mistake, they had to start over from the beginning.

Before this experiment, the participants had been split into two groups: the first group were told to write a page about a deep personal value, such as integrity or honesty, that was important to them. The second group were told to write about something they didn't care about. What happened? In the second group, the lack of approval or acceptance from the panel caused a cortisol stress response. The group who had written about a personal value prior to the interview remained calm. Their cortisol levels were the same before and after the event. This is a good indication that focusing on our core values can help us to stay centred in the best version of ourselves. Give it a try!

If you enjoyed thinking about your values, I have two more exercises that will consolidate these concepts in your mind, and help you find ways to incorporate your *ikigai* every day.

Prioritising your values

This is an exercise originally devised by therapist Tobias Lundgren, and more recently adapted by psychologist Dr Julie Smith into a values 'star' in her book *Why Has Nobody Told Me This Before?*[40] To keep things even simpler, I have devised a values triangle. Add each of your current top three values to the points on the triangle, and decide, on a scale of 1 to 10, how your life currently matches your values of importance. If your value is 'family' and you are working hard on a lot of business projects and seeing less of the kids than you would like, you might mark this at 5/10. If your value is 'health' and you're cooking balanced meals and moving your body and feeling good, you might mark this as 9/10. You can then mark each value on the triangle by that number. As you join the dots, you can see the shape of your triangle, and the areas that are uneven are those you can give your attention.

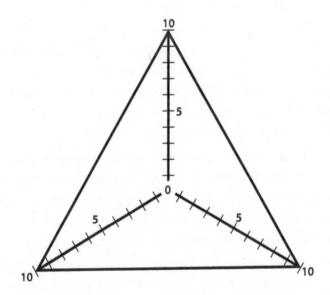

The values triangle. Simply add a dot to represent each of your top three values to the diagram, and join the dots to see the shape of your triangle. This will help you visualise where you want to focus most attention moving forwards, to even out your triangle.

Code words exercise

Sometimes we need a personal example to ignite our imagination and make our most important values even clearer to us. My husband, storytelling expert and author Richard Newman, talked about the concept of creating 'code words' in his book *Lift Your Impact*.[41] In the book, he shared the idea that finding a phrase unique to you can immediately connect you to your values, which can in turn create more of an emotional impact. He gave an example of his number-one value which is 'being a good father' and then he asked himself, 'What one word or phrase describes this well?' The answer he found was unique to him: 'polar bears'. When our children were younger, they invented a game where Richard would get down on all fours, with one of our sons climbing on his back and the other hiding underneath him. They would then patrol the wilderness to find food, shelter, play, laugh and enjoy quality time together. For him, this word and memory truly embodied his core value, and reminded him of it much more powerfully.

For me, one of my core values was compassion. I realised that recognising suffering in others and then taking steps to help relieve it was the main purpose behind my career choice. Compassion is also the reason I decided I'd enjoy a 100 per cent plant-based diet, rather than a mostly plant-based diet. Compassion is a tangible expression of love. When I underwent my Jikiden Reiki training, I learned more about a fascinating deity venerated across eastern Asia in Buddhist and Taoist faiths, known in Sanskrit as Padmapani ('born of the lotus') and originally worshipped in male as well as female forms. She is 'Quan Yin' (or 'Guan Yin'), the goddess of compassion, and her paintings and statues can be found throughout many parts of the world in temples, shops and homes. She really did seem to embody the value in a specific way. So I chose her as my code word. I have a small collection of statues depicting her in my home, and seeing the statues from time to time, along with repeating my code word each morning, happens to be a good reminder of the value of compassion throughout my day.

What are your code words? Try to think of one for each of the values you identified on page 97. Write them below.

Value 1:
Code word for value 1:

Value 2:
Code word for value 2:

Value 3:
Code word for value 3:

You can write these code words somewhere you'll see them a lot; maybe on a sticky note on your bathroom mirror, fridge or bedside table, or you could have an image of one of your code words on your phone's home screen. You could also write them at the front of your diary or journal. Seeing these words when you wake up will anchor you to them and help remind you why they are important. As you prepare for sleep and your mind is releasing the day, seeing your code words could also inspire thoughts and dreams that help you feel good about how you're going to feel tomorrow. Give it a go. It's a powerful way to connect with yourself every day.

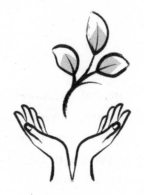

Outside

In this chapter I want you to consider two things. First and foremost, how often you go outside – and I don't mean popping to the shops, or your commute to work (and sitting in the car doesn't count)! How often do you take a moment to go outside to enjoy the natural world around you?

We will look at all the benefits we know that nature can bring to our health and distil that evidence into some simple daily habits for you to try.

I also want you to consider your home setup. This is because there might be changes indoors, using the healing power of plants, that you can make that could dramatically improve your health. You might not realise how your living space can impact your health, but I have seen so many benefits for my patients from making changes to their lifestyle and home environment. As we have discussed at the start of this book, what we experience, how we live and what we eat – they all impact our health. I am an advocate for a plant-powered life as much as a plant-powered diet, and I want to show you why . . .

Let me tell you about a patient, Alan, who came to see me after months of feeling burned out. He had been working from home since the pandemic started and his mental health and his sleep patterns had deteriorated badly. He was answering emails and going to online meetings without breaks, and finding himself struggling so much that he couldn't remember important information. He began falling behind in his work. Alan was so tired, yet he couldn't sleep, and was so wired yet unable to focus.

One morning, as he opened his email inbox, he collapsed and

began to cry. It was at this point of crisis that his wife encouraged him to book an appointment with me.

Listening to his routine, it became clear that despite a healthy diet, he was struggling to feel energised. He was in a room without natural light for most of the day. He didn't have time for a walk and spent hours sitting at his desk, not moving.

I suggested he start small – I asked him to find a picture of a nature scene that he really liked and put it on his wall where he could turn to see it from his desk. I encouraged him to take two five-minute tea breaks, during which he also did some simple stretches and star jumps, outside, in his garden, with bare feet.

When I checked in with him a month later, he had noticed a profound difference in his wellbeing. He no longer felt panicked. He found his ability to focus on productive work had improved. He felt able to increase his outdoor time to take a short walk around the block during his lunch break. He was sleeping better and found himself less irritable. He felt he could create clearer boundaries between his work time and personal time through the day. On an annual leave day, he felt comfortable putting on his out-of-office email response and didn't feel the need to check his emails. On this occasion, a 'green prescription' worked far better than a pill!

The evidence showing the restorative power of the natural world is abundant and exciting. Let's look at the key ways it could help you too.

The benefits of sunlight

In understanding why Alan got so much benefit from just a hand-ful of changes to his day, let's start with an experience that will hopefully resonate with most people. Have you noticed how the sun makes you feel better? I find I am definitely more peaceful, focused and productive when I have had my dose of sunlight. Just as plants absorb and metabolise sunlight, we do too. We must have enough light for optimal health.

The benefits of being outside are vast. But we know that the risk of all types of skin cancer rises with excess sun exposure, especially with burning. Later I will discuss how to get the balance right when it comes to being under the sun's rays. But first, why could it benefit us to spend some time outdoors and in the sunshine? Researchers have found that the health benefits of sun exposure for our hearts (in terms of lowering blood pressure and cardiovascular mortality) increase with more time in the sun, independent of vitamin D supplementation.[1] This could be because when the sun touches our skin, nitric oxide is released (which also happens when we eat leafy green vegetables, by the way!) and this has a positive effect on our blood pressure. As a reminder, maintaining a healthy blood pressure is important for cutting the risk of heart disease and strokes, which are a much more common cause of death than skin cancer.[2]

When the sun hits our skin, it also triggers our body to make vitamin D – this is the only way the body can make vitamin D – a fat-soluble vitamin and hormone that has a variety of functions. Perhaps the most important one being the regulation of the absorption of calcium and phosphate in the body. Getting a sufficient amount of vitamin D, sometimes called the 'sunshine vitamin', is important for the growth and development of bones throughout our lives.[3] In children, a lack of vitamin D can cause rickets and in adults, it can result in osteomalacia, a condition where the bones become softer, leading to pain and risk of fractures. Women who have missed more than a few months of periods in their fertile years are more likely to develop thinning of the bones at, or even before, the menopause (osteopenia). Vitamin D therapy is a key part of helping to strengthen bones to prevent osteoporosis as well.

There are vitamin D receptors all over our body, and so it is also thought to be responsible for a number of other important jobs too. It seems to play a critical role in regulating our mood, warding off seasonal affective disorder or SAD (see below), balancing our immune system, lowering our risk of diabetes, and even reducing our risk of certain cancers.[4] Incredibly, one study found that vitamin D helped brain function. It looked at vitamin D levels in more than 1,700 men and women in England who were aged 65 and over. The study discovered that the lower the participants' vitamin D levels, the more negatively impacted their performance was in a series of mental tests.[5] Given the many roles of vitamin D, supplementation is important for many of us, who live more indoor lifestyles and may not make enough of this important vitamin.

The sun is nature's antidepressant

Have you ever described someone as having a 'sunny disposition'? A blast of sunshine increases the levels of the mood-lifting endorphin serotonin.[6] When our levels of this chemical rise, we feel happy, energised and alert. Without enough exposure to sunlight, levels of serotonin drop.[7] People who work shifts or long hours where they do not get outside may be more at risk of suffering from SAD, a depressive illness influenced by changing seasonal light levels and frequencies.[8,9] SAD is often treated with artificial light from lamps that are designed to mimic natural sunlight.

Our mental health can also be adversely affected by a disrupted circadian rhythm (which is the internal body clock that regulates our sleep–wake cycle over a 24-hour period).[10,11] We know that sleep deprivation can induce mania in people with bipolar disorder (more on sleep deprivation in the sleep chapter on page 253), but some evidence suggests a disrupted circadian rhythm can also play a part.[12] A small, randomised placebo-controlled study involving a group of 32 patients with bipolar disorder in Norway, showed that the use of glasses that block blue light, in addition to therapy, improved their mental health and reduced relapse rates.[13] Why is this important? Morning light sets our sleep–wake rhythm, and there are different frequencies of light from the sun at different times of day. At midday, there is more blue light and ultraviolet light. Then as sunset approaches, the balance shifts again to higher amounts of red and infrared light. Blue light is also emitted by devices like smartphones, tablets, computers and TV screens, which can therefore mimic the effects of midday light on our eyes and brains.

Although more research is needed, I believe this finding is relevant for all of us, given the clear link between low mood and insomnia, and low mood and light deprivation.

Why does spending time outside help us sleep better at night? Exposure to photons as part of normal sunlight, within the first half hour or so of the sunrise, offers the ideal balance of UV and infrared light, encouraging the body to release the feel-good endorphin serotonin.[14] It follows that getting outside soon after we wake up (even on an overcast or rainy day) for just a few minutes is the perfect wake-up reset. This is such a simple tip to add to your routine, especially if you have trouble falling asleep.

At night, melatonin, the chemical in your brain that makes you feel drowsy and fall asleep, is made in the body from serotonin (so what you get from the sunrise helps you relax at sunset). This messenger, sometimes called the 'sleep hormone', not only makes us fall asleep but also synchronises our internal body clock and improves the quality of our sleep.[15] This, in turn, helps to regulate our immune system, support cardiac health and regulate our appetite, among other things.[16-18]

Our sleep–wake cycles have evolved over thousands of years, from when our ancestors' days began with the rising sun. Today, we are constantly exposed to bright light, with lightbulbs, TVs, smartphones, tablets and laptops, and as mentioned above, our bodies can misinterpret this light as sunlight.[19] The constant blue light confuses our pineal gland, preventing it from making enough melatonin to help us sleep. That is why it is so important to switch off from devices in the evening at least an hour before you go to bed, so your internal body clock is less affected.[20]

Our eyes do not just 'see' the world; they also transmit important information to our brains about what hormones we should be producing and when. Our brains respond to blue light in a remarkable way. Specialised retinal ganglion cells, a type of neuron located near the inner surface of the retina of the eye, detect daylight. These stimulate the brain, which lets the pineal gland know to make more melatonin.[21]

We don't yet know the long-term effects of being exposed to blue light all day and all night. As blue light is one of the few colours of the light spectrum that is able to penetrate to the back of the retina – unlike UV light, for example – the concern is that it may increase the risk of degenerative eye disorders involving the retina, with prolonged exposure over time.[22-26] More research needs to be done. While we wait for that, I urge you to consider how much blue light your body is exposed to, and consider ways to reduce it at least an hour before bedtime.

The interactions between sunlight, vitamin D, serotonin and our circadian rhythms are complex. Research is even showing that our gut bacteria are affected negatively by disrupted sleep patterns (and jet lag).[27] I'll cover more about this in the sleep chapter on page 253. We cannot live well when we are separated from the world outside. Our bodies are connected to the sun.

How to enjoy the sun safely

What is a healthy dose of sunlight? While there are benefits to exposure to sunlight, it is not without its own health risks. Overexposure to the sun's ultraviolet (UV) rays can lead to a risk of burning in the short term, and skin cancer in the long term.[28] This is the big dilemma. A number of studies (including large populations of people as well as cell studies) actually show vitamin D reduces the risk and the outcomes of internal cancers.[29] So how can we get the balance right between reducing the risk of skin cancer and having enough sun to get the vitamin D we need to reduce the risk of other cancers?

Here is the key advice we need to consider: due to skin cancer risks, dermatologists generally recommend spending time in the shade between 11am and 3pm (when the sun is strongest) between March and October, and taking particular care with children.

However, between 11am and 3pm is also the most efficient time to experience the most intense UVB rays for vitamin D production – which, as we know, is a vital vitamin for our bodies to function optimally. Vitamin D can only be made by UVB exposure.[30] What is the difference between UVA and UVB light? Ultraviolet A (UVA) has a longer wavelength, and is associated with skin aging, and with tanning. UVA light is less intense than UVB, which is associated with skin burning, but over 90 per cent of UV light from the sun is in the form of UVA. It is also present constantly in daylight hours throughout the year. UVB light, on the other hand, fluctuates throughout the day and has a shorter wavelength. You can't get the same level of UVB needed to keep your vitamin D levels topped up by sitting near a sunny window, indoors. You need to be outside.

It is hard to get enough light to make good amounts of vitamin D when we live in northerly latitudes, but timing is key. One study looking at countries such as Poland and the UK found midday exposure to be the most efficient time of day to synthesize vitamin D from the sun.[31] Tanning beds are not a good idea; the UVA radiation emitted from them can be up to three times more intense than the UVA in natural sunlight, and they have been associated with increased risk of early onset melanoma.[32] All of this data points to there being some benefit in spending some time in the sun between 11am and 3pm.

So what should you do?

Sun salutations

It's so easy to be overzealous in countries like the UK, where we have an inclination to see the sun, strip off and end up looking like a lobster. But we could also benefit from a different kind of sun safety than staying out of the sun altogether. Try short bursts in the midday sun instead.

For pale skin, around 13 minutes of midday sunlight in summer months, three times a week, is enough to make adequate amounts of vitamin D.[33] Try exposing your arms and legs for a short walk, sitting in the garden with a cup of tea or some gentle stretching outside before lunch.

If you have a darker skin tone, you'll need anywhere between 30 minutes and three hours more sunshine to make enough vitamin D.[34-37] I would have liked to add specific advice on sun-exposure times for different skin tones, but sadly I could not find that information. This is where more research is needed. I think it is also worth getting a blood test to check your blood levels of vitamin D, so you know your baseline and can supplement where necessary.

If you are outside for longer periods, I do encourage you to cover up, wear sunglasses and a hat and apply sunscreen on exposed areas to protect your skin from cancer. I recommend using a sunscreen that does not contain ingredients like oxybenzone, octinoxate, enzacamene (4-MBC) and zinc oxide. These can be harmful to aquatic life and corals (which can enter the sea via our sewage systems as well as swimming).[38,39] Instead, opt for a sunscreen that uses titanium dioxide, octocrylene, octisalate, avobenzone, octyl triazone (Uvinul T) ecamsule (Mexoryl SX) or Drometrizole trisiloxane (Mexotyl XL). These ingredients have been shown to cause minimal or no harm.

Look for sunscreens that are gentle to sensitive skin, and that will protect you from both **UVB** and **UVA** radiation. The words 'broad spectrum' and 'full spectrum' will indicate coverage for both types of radiation. Stay safe, and instead of fearing the sun, let's appreciate its power and enjoy it wisely.

Tips for a safe sun-loving lifestyle

* ❀ **Go outside as soon as you wake, or as soon as it's light**, whichever comes first. A few minutes can make a big difference to reset your sleep–wake cycle.
* ❀ **Note in your diary or phone how often you got outside last week** – if it's less than 30 minutes a day, is there a way you could get outside more?
* ❀ **Blue light-free bedtime!** Cut the screens, start to use low lights (or salt lamps) instead of harsh overhead

lights as the evening draws in. Could you benefit from blue light-blocking glasses in the evening?

* **Consider checking your vitamin D** status and supplementing if you need to.
* **Sun in the middle of the day can be most efficient for vitamin D production** – can you aim for short bursts of sun exposure and then a sensible cover-up?
* **If you're out in the sun for long periods, to reduce risk of burning and skin cancer, you can stick to the shade**, cover up and wear sunglasses and sunscreen.
* **Try mineral sunscreen for sensitive skin** and to avoid certain chemicals harmful to aquatic life.

Nature really can heal

When we are 'in our heads', we tend to be thinking about the past and the future, rather than the present moment – the time we are actually living in. It can be hard to get perspective and see a way through. Perhaps we cannot 'see the wood for the trees'.

If that's you, let's take a moment right now.

Close your eyes and breathe out – pushing the air out of your lungs. Don't breathe in just yet. Try pushing the air out of your lungs a couple more times – expel the old air from your lungs. While you do this, can you imagine you are surrounded by trees? Imagine the sounds of the birds singing in the trees, imagine the smell of the leaves, imagine the sunlight peeking through the branches. Breathe deeply, filling your lungs with oxygen. How do you feel?

Nature imagery tends to help us feel calm and relaxed. And it turns out being in nature can also have an array of physical benefits. A team of researchers found that people who spend time in green spaces have a significantly reduced risk of a number of chronic diseases, including reduced risk of type 2 diabetes and heart disease, preterm birth, stress, and high blood pressure.[40-43] Alas, the exact mechanisms of why this happens are unknown! But we have a few clues to work with:

- We know that being outside is an important way to synthesise vitamin D.
- UV light has an effect on the skin microbiome in modulating our immune system.
- The photons of light on the back of our eyes (retina) can stimulate the production of serotonin, some of which will convert to melatonin, the sleep hormone, which helps our body to achieve restorative sleep that is vital for our immune system and physiology.
- Being outside may also mean we are socialising.

In addition, trees and plants emit airborne phytoncides, antimicrobial organic compounds, which protect them from germs. We breathe in these compounds when we spend time in nature, and our bodies respond by increasing the amount of a type of white blood cell called natural killer cells (or NK cells).[44] These cells are critical to our immune systems because they help our bodies fight disease. One study showed that men who took two 80-minute guided walks on the same day in a forest setting had around a 50 per cent spike in NK cells compared to completing the guided walks in an urban setting.[45] Another study showed that women who logged four hours in the forest on two consecutive days also had around a 40 per cent increase in cancer-fighting white blood cells.[43-44] Evergreens, including conifers, spruce, pine and cedar, are the largest producers of phytoncides.

When we are outside, physiological stress is also reduced and both blood pressure and heart rate are lowered. One study monitored 280 participants in 24 walking groups in Japan. One group walked through the forest and the other group walked through the city. The results showed that when walking through the forest, participants had lower cortisol rates, lower pulse rates, greater parasympathetic nervous system activity and lower blood pressure compared to those walking through urban areas.[47,48]

Dr Qing Li is one of the world's leading experts in forest medicine, and has conducted many studies in this area, including the ones I mention above. He has really brought the traditional Japanese practice of *shinrin-yoku* into the public consciousness internationally. *Shinrin-yoku* roughly translates as 'forest bathing', meaning to soak up the sights, sounds and smells of the natural setting. In Japan it is taken very seriously and has become a cornerstone of preventative health and healing.

For those who live in cities and towns and don't have easy access to the countryside, please do not be discouraged. A walk around your local park (the more trees and plants the better) during your lunch hour can make a huge difference. It is harder to remember that we are a part of nature, and how it can make us feel good, when we don't have easy access to it.

Breathing the biome

With every breath we take, we draw upon the oxygen produced by plants. When we head outside in nature, one of the first things we do almost automatically is take a big breath of fresh air. Our bodies rely on our gut microbes – those trillions of bugs in our digestive systems – to help digest our food, regulate our immunity and produce essential vitamins. But there is a growing area of research around how the air we breathe influences our gut microbiome too. If the air we breathe is polluted, airborne pollutants can play a role in the onset of chronic disease.

According to the World Health Organization (WHO), air pollution is the largest environmental risk factor for human disease.[49] Over 7 million people die from air-pollution-related causes *each year* (that's more people than died of COVID-19 during the pandemic).[50] This is because long-term exposure to air pollution can cause or contribute to long-term conditions such as heart disease, lung disease and lung cancer, which can all affect our life expectancy. In the UK, air pollution is the largest environmental risk to public health.[51]

It is also true that polluted air has the ability to carry pathogens more easily; pollution is likely to have carried viruses including bird flu, measles, foot-and-mouth disease and SARS-CoV-2.[51]

Research suggests that black carbon, a large component of air pollution, changes how bacteria grow, and helps them to form biofilms. A biofilm is a slimy substance that forms when bacteria stick to living surfaces (e.g. tissues like the lungs). The glue-like biofilm increases the bacteria's chances of survival in the lining of airways and their ability to resist antibiotics.[52]

This is why, if my patients have respiratory problems and can afford to, I will often suggest buying a HEPA air filter for their home, and ask them to consider walking routes that minimise their exposure to high-density traffic wherever possible.[53]

It was once widely accepted that the lungs were a sterile environment, and that there were no microbes or bacteria present. Now we know that the surfaces of the airways have their own community of microbes, which may be disrupted in common lung diseases like chronic obstructive pulmonary disease (COPD) and asthma.[54] One of the latest areas of scientific research is the importance of microbes within respiratory health.

Can we develop and maintain a healthy lung microbiome?

As with the gut microbiome, colonisation begins during and after birth. It is thought that living in rural areas encourages a greater diversity of gut, lung and skin microbes, which is one of the reasons why there is a lower rate of asthma and allergies in rural populations.[55] From early research, one of the easiest ways to naturally increase microbe diversity in our lungs is simply by being exposed to different types of beneficial bacteria from being outside in nature. Being around pets is another way to do this.

Tips for breathing the biome

- **Daily green time:** can you spend your lunchtime in a green space, walking among trees and spend some time near trees three times a week? Inner-city parks and green spaces are ideal for this.
- **Defra's UK air website provides forecasts and current air-pollution levels, while in the US the Air Quality Index (AQI) is useful.** There are free air-quality apps you can download in many countries; what's available in your area?
- **Limiting exercise in high-pollution areas** or during times of high pollution helps, especially if you are prone to asthma.
- **If there is highly polluted outdoor air, close doors and windows that face a busy street** during congested periods.
- **Consider getting a HEPA air filter** for your home.

The healing power of water

How do you feel when you are by the sea? As well as being in the green of nature, there is also a unique feeling of peace and serenity that we derive from being near water. It is the essence of life, after all, with water making up around 70 per cent of our planet's surface and 55–70 per cent of our bodies.

I grew up living by the sea, and my walks along the seafront – in all weather conditions – were a weekend treat that kept me going all week. I still relish the sound and sight of the waves crashing against the sand, and seeing the power of the waves, the tides and the seasons playing out on the water.

Blue mind science is the study of aquatic environments and how they benefit us. This idea was pioneered by US marine biologist Wallace J Nichols. He believes we all have a 'blue mind' that is triggered when we are in, or near, water because it induces a meditative state that makes us happier, calmer, healthier and more creative.[56] In our modern world, we are bombarded with anxiety-inducing sensory input, a state that Nichols calls the 'red mind'. Our brains need time to rest and recover, and the sight and sound of water is much easier to process than modern elements of daily life. The same is true of fractals, small-scale examples of geometric designs, when we witness them in nature; both trigger a relaxation response in our brains (for more on fractals, see page 126). All our senses are engaged when we are by water or can hear water, and this allows our brains to process thoughts in a different way.

The health effects of 'blue spaces' are an emerging topic of study for an increasing number of professionals. BlueHealth, a pan-European research initiative, has been looking at the links between environment, climate and health – and the best ways to use water to boost the wellbeing of people in urban areas. The researchers noted that many of the benefits, including stress reduction, are similar to those reaped by being in green spaces.[57]

As with everything in the natural world, it is free and accessible to everyone. Fortunately, you do not need to live by the sea to feel the benefits. One study measured the heart rates and blood pressure of people while they viewed an empty tank of water, a partially filled aquarium tank with fish and plants, and then a fully stocked tank with double the number of animal species. The study found that just by looking at tanks of water, including the empty water tank, people's blood pressure and heart rates were both lowered – although the therapeutic benefits increased as more biodiversity was added.[58] So, whether you use a picture of the sea as your screen saver or commit to visit the beach as often as you can, it can boost your mental health and happiness.

How to benefit from a blue mind

- ❀ **If you're lucky enough to live near the sea, carve out some time to go** and visit as often as you can!
- ❀ **In urban settings, find a lake or pond in a local park –** even a water fountain can provide some water therapy.
- ❀ **The flowing water in a river can be very calming.** If you live near a river, make time for river walks.
- ❀ **Can you combine movement with water?** Rowing, kayaking, paddleboarding, surfing and, of course, swimming are great ways to connect with water.
- ❀ **Can you bring water to your home space?** It doesn't have to be a fish tank; even a water feature on a balcony or terrace could provide the healing sound of running water at home.

❀ **Images of water are powerful too;** do you have a favourite painting or photo of the sea? Pop it up on the wall, or add a water scene to your computer's home screen.

Cold-water therapy works

I love the feeling of being invigorated after a dip in a cold lake or sea. I remember jumping in a lake in Vienna in January (my husband thought I was mad!) and wading into the Irish sea in my bikini at sunrise in February. Both times, it felt like the last thing I wanted to do, but afterwards, the rush left me with a warm glow for the rest of the day. And there is a reason for that. Cold-water therapy – whether it's a quick outdoor swim in cold water, a post-workout ice bath, or a brisk cold shower – could benefit our health in a number of ways. Research shows cold-water therapy can reduce post-workout muscle soreness and help you cool down more quickly after overheating from a sweaty workout.[59]

Small studies have reported mental health benefits of regular cold-water immersion,[60] and proponents such as Wim Hof, who devised The Wim Hof Method, showed in a series of controlled experiments how a combination of breathing techniques and cold-water immersion improved the immune response when the body was exposed to doses of potentially harmful bacterial pathogens.[61] Some advocates also say it can improve your sleep and sharpen your mental focus, although I do want to be clear that more research is needed.

If you decide to give cold-water immersion a try, always go with someone else if you plan to swim in open water. Heart attacks during open-water swimming can happen, and you can have too much of a good thing, risking hypothermia. Immersion can affect your blood pressure and heart rate, so if you have a pre-existing heart condition, it can cause significant cardiac stress. Much like with exercise, a bit of 'hormetic' stress is good for your body and metabolism, you just need to know how much is right for you. Start slowly, and be gentle with your body.

For a safer outdoor immersion, have a short swim – is there a lido or swimming pond near you? There are no known benefits for staying in very cold water for long periods of time. Once you are out of the water, immediately put on a hat and gloves and aim to get out of wet clothes quickly. Drink a nice warm drink from a flask and have a sweet snack (sugar can help elevate body temperature) and walk briskly to a warm place. Avoid taking an immediate hot shower as the sudden change in blood flow could cause you to faint – and can give you painful toes . . . I know from personal experience!

Make your own ice bath!

An at-home way to experience cold-water immersion: add ice to a cold-water bath until the temperature is between 10°C and 15°C. If you can, stay submerged for up to 15 minutes before getting out and warming up.

Cold-shower therapy

The simplest way for most of us to experience cold-water therapy, if you don't have access to safe swimming spots or don't fancy an ice bath just yet, is to have a cold shower.

The largest study looking at the benefits of cold showers on the human body took place in the Netherlands, with over 3,000 participants, and lasted for a month, with a further two-month follow-up period. Researchers found that the group who took a warm shower, followed by a cold shower of 30, 60 or 90 seconds, took

29 per cent fewer self-reported sick days in the three-month winter trial period than those who had a warm-water shower only.[62]

Why not give it a try and see how it impacts you?

Tips for introducing cold-water therapy

- ✸ **Start off small** – 15 seconds of cold water after your warm shower – then build up your tolerance over time. You might find it takes your breath away at first, so remember to breathe deeply during the cold shower, starting with pushing the air out of your lungs first.
- ✸ **Every little helps.** The study in the Netherlands showed benefits in as little as 30 seconds, but research suggests benefits can wane after three minutes.
- ✸ **Go straight to a cold shower** if you've just finished working out. If you go to a gym with a sauna, try cold-water immersion after using the sauna for even more hormetic stress and potential benefits.

Have you heard of 'grounding'?

My kids dislike going outside barefoot, unless it's sunny and warm! But for me, there is something really special about the feeling of grass beneath my feet and between my toes. Grounding, sometimes referred to as 'earthing', is as simple as walking barefoot outdoors and/or using inexpensive grounding equipment indoors, e.g. a 'grounding mat' while sleeping or sitting. But is this just tree-hugging mumbo-jumbo or is there actually something in it we could benefit from physiologically?

Generations ago, people tended to spend more time outside – working on farms, in domestic environments or in physical jobs.

There were also fewer physical barriers between the human body and the earth's natural surfaces. We did not have carpeted homes and offices. In the last hundred years or so, we also tend to wear rubber- or plastic-soled shoes. Both of these materials act as insulators, which means an electrical charge can't flow through them. Why is this relevant?

All modern electrical systems, from large power grids to homes and factories, and even the electrical appliances we use every day, are connected to the earth for stability and safety. Think about a plug; there is a copper earth wire connected to the case, which provides a low-resistance path to the ground. This protects you from an electric shock by providing a path for a fault current to flow to the earth.

The surface of the earth is affected by lightning strikes, solar radiation, and other atmospheric dynamics. These charged environmental phenomena give the land and water a continuously renewed supply of electrons, which makes the earth a natural source of negative electrical charge. The theory behind grounding for humans is that the electrons from the earth can have a positive impact on our bodies.[63] Compare it to the health benefits we get from berries, which contain electrons that mop up positively charged free radicals in our bodies and combat oxidative stress. Similarly, contact with the ground can be a form of 'electric nutrition'.[64,65]

Research in this area is still quite scant; there is nowhere near the volume of data we have on the role of nutrition for health, for example, but I think the data looks interesting and shows correlations between practising grounding and the relief of a range of ailments.[64,66,67]

In one very small study, blood samples were taken before and after grounding, and researchers looked for changes in blood cell viscosity, or 'stickiness'. Low viscosity is important for cardiovascular health because it helps to maintain a steady flow of blood cells in the vessels. The results showed that grounding significantly reduced viscosity and clustering of red blood cells.[68] This is important as, in the long term, it could reduce the risk of cardiovascular disease. Three of the subjects were also experiencing pain, and two of these reported that their pain was gone after two hours of grounding, with the third reporting that her pain had nearly gone.

Another small study recruited people who were suffering from sleep disturbances and chronic pain. Half slept on grounding mats (a simple mat that usually connects via a wire to the ground port of an electrical outlet in your home, which mimics the effect of lying directly on the ground), while the other half slept on placebo mats. Those who were grounded reported a reduction in pain, better sleep and symptomatic improvements and relief from conditions including asthma and other respiratory conditions, as well as rheumatoid arthritis, premenstrual syndrome (PMS), sleep apnoea, and hypertension.[69,70] I see these findings as hopeful that grounding could be an effective, simple and completely free treatment to help reduce pain and improve sleep. These are very small studies, and we need to know more. Listening to people who have felt calmer after trying grounding, I wonder if it helps shift the body from the sympathetic nervous system's fight-or-flight stress response towards the parasympathetic nervous system's 'rest and recovery' state as well.

Grounding exercise

Do you know the scene from the movie *Pretty Woman*, in which Julia Roberts's character is trying to encourage the workaholic lawyer, played by Richard Gere, to live a little? She tells him to take off his shoes and walk barefoot on the grass.

Take off your shoes and socks. Go into your garden or do this in your local park for a few minutes every day. It's a quick and simple energy booster.

Even better, if you are near water, take a barefoot stroll along the water's edge at the beach or on the dewy grass and see how you feel. The contact with the water and earth is believed to be a more powerful experience. I love it. Try it for yourself.

Simple ways to try grounding:

❀ Do some gardening, without gloves or barefoot, so you can feel the soil.
❀ Have a nap on the grass.
❀ Exercise outside barefoot.
❀ Rest against a tree for a while.
❀ Touch natural environments, including rocks, plants and trees, with bare hands.
❀ Immerse yourself in a natural body of water such as an ocean, stream or lake.
❀ Look online for at-home grounding devices for your bed or chair, which can give you the benefits of grounding while you sleep or relax on the sofa.

Restorative nature patterns

We are innately visual creatures. We know through research that simply looking at natural scenes can have an impact on how our autonomic nervous systems respond to stress.[71] I have scenes of nature in my consultation room, and over the years many patients have commented on how calming it was to look at them as they were having their blood pressure taken! This can also be true for hospital settings. One study showed that patients whose hospital window overlooked natural settings recorded shorter recovery times, required less medication and noted their hospital stay was more positive than those who did not have a nature view.[72] There are many ideas about why this could be, but one of the most interesting possible explanations is the effect of fractals.

Fractals are patterns that repeat themselves. These repeating patterns can be big or small, and in the natural world fractals surround us. The most obvious example of fractals in nature is the branch of a tree. Each branch is a copy of the one that came before it. In our own bodies, our lungs have fractals repeating into smaller units, much like a tree branch does. Fractals in nature include clouds, seashells, trees, flowers, snowflakes, leaves, plants, rivers, coastlines and mountains. Our brains have developed to look at fractals and process them quickly.[73]

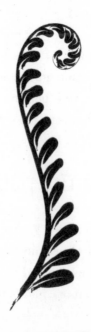

Scientists say that just looking at fractals can lower our stress by up to 60 per cent because of a physiological resonance in the eye that takes just a few seconds.[74] Once I started to notice them, it took my nature gazing to whole new levels! It also reminded me why I used to love shell and fossil collecting so much as a child. The patterns I'd see used to fascinate me. Try it for yourself.

A positive mental-energy boost

The concept of biophilia – a love of the world around us – suggests we have a fundamental need for contact with nature.[75] The word originates from the Greek word *philia*, meaning 'love of'. It literally means a love of life or living things. The phrase was first used by Edward O. Wilson in his book *Biophilia*, published in 1984, and the biophilia hypothesis supports the idea that humans are healthier when they are connected to nature.[76] This concept has filtered into town planning, green design and eco-friendly architecture as well.[77]

It is abundantly clear from a number of well-designed studies over the last few years that biophilia now also has a scientific basis.[78] Connecting with nature can have a profound effect on our mental health.[79] During one study, two groups were asked to walk for 90 minutes a day, one group in a natural area and the other in a high-traffic urban setting. Researchers measured the group's heart and respiration rates, conducted brain scans and asked them to fill out questionnaires. While there was little difference in physiological conditions, there were significant differences in the brain. Those people who walked in nature showed reduced activity in the sub-genual prefrontal cortex, a region of the brain associated with rumination, a key factor in depression.[80] The study also showed that being in nature helps us to regulate our emotions and encourages us to think outwards about the environment, rather than get caught in negative thought patterns.

Could there be benefits other than to our mood? Countless studies over the years have shown the link between exposure to nature and an increased sense of wellbeing and energy. One series of experiments showed that being in nature does actually make us feel 'more alive' by boosting feelings of both physical and mental energy by nearly 40 per cent.[81] The sense of increased vitality went beyond the energising effects of physical activity or social interactions. Participants described the therapeutic experience as 'fuel for the soul'. How lovely is that?

One study from Harvard University observed over 100,000 people and found that those living in the greenest areas had a 12 per cent lower mortality rate, compared with those living in built-up areas.[82] This is why it is something that medical practitioners should take note of too. If you live in a city or urban area, please don't be discouraged. Bringing the power of nature into our lives is possible in so many ways that don't involve having to move. Remember, even looking at images of nature, or tending to a pot of fresh herbs on your windowsill count towards bring nature benefits into your life.

Luckily, the power of nature and connection (see page 80) are being recognised by healthcare organisations now. 'Social prescribing' is an effective way for doctors to refer their patients to health-promoting, community-based support.[83] It has become very popular here in the UK, and a recent report by the Global Social Prescribing Alliance shows it is a way of providing holistic healthcare that has also been adopted in many countries around the world.[84] Social prescribing links people to local social support groups, and brings people together with others who live in their community. I am thrilled to report that many of these social prescribing activities revolve around the natural world; park runs and community gardens have become more popular, and walking groups are popping up across the country too.

Visual biology and nature gazing

When stress becomes chronic, we can experience visual symptoms such as eye strain and blurry vision caused by higher levels of cortisol and adrenaline circulating in the bloodstream.[85] If you experience this, or even simple eye strain from spending too long looking at a screen, research shows shifting your focus to something further away (ideally involving a nature view) can be calming for the eyes and brain.[86] Dry eyes and digital eye strain are more common with increasing use of smartphones and technology, especially since the 2020 pandemic.[87] A simple way to mitigate this? Try regularly shifting your focus from your computer screen to looking out of the window, at the horizon or up into the trees. Maybe go for a walk if you can't see any from your desk!

If you can't spare the time to get outside, simply allow your eyes to shift focus. You can widen your gaze, relax and become aware of what you can see in your peripheral vision. This allows you to take in more of your surroundings. This technique helps reduce stress because our eyes are linked to our autonomic nervous system. So by allowing a simple shift of visual focus, we can also gain a higher tolerance for stressful situations.

This simple 'hack' can work wherever you are, and is helpful in a stressful presentation or a boardroom meeting – or even at a soft play area with arguing children and high levels of ambient noise! Being outside can allow this gaze-widening effect more instinctively, which is a great way to combine nature and biology to boost our mood.[88]

Nature-based health tips

We do not need a huge amount of time in nature to feel its bene-fits.[89] I encourage my patients to try 20 to 30 minutes outside in daylight, four or five times a week, which really can make all the difference. The key to any habit change is to make it part of your daily routine. Whether this is tending to plants and flowers in the garden, taking a stroll in the park or woodlands, or being around animals in their natural habitats, natural environments can make us feel more peaceful and connected.

Do any of these ideas resonate with you and could they bring you joy?

- ❀ Go for a walk and ask yourself: what can you see, hear and smell? Practise paying more attention to the plants and wildlife around you to feel their positive effects.
- ❀ Exercise outdoors on your own or with other people – in the garden, if you have one, or in the local park.
- ❀ Can you make time to go into the countryside and make a longer experience of a walk?
- ❀ Try growing flowers, houseplants or even your own vegetables and herbs – you can do this in the smallest garden, a pot or window box or inside. Bring nature into your home.
- ❀ Look up at the stars at night when you are brushing your teeth before bed.
- ❀ Eat outdoors – can you take your lunch to a local green space?
- ❀ Check out the community gardens in your area. Do you have the time to share an allotment and grow food with other people?

❀ Working at your computer, tablet, phone or laptop? Take one or two minutes every half an hour to purposely shift your gaze and allow more awareness of what is in your peripheral vision.

❀ Can you have an image of nature next to your desk, or on your screen saver?

❀ Notice fractals. If you are in a park or forest, look up at the tree branches. If you're at the beach, look down for shells and patterns in the rocks.

❀ Go back to page 112 for safe, sun-loving lifestyle tips.

❀ See page 115 for suggestions about breathing the biome.

❀ Incorporate grounding into your daily routine (see page 122).

Nature therapy indoors

I want to now turn our attention inside, and look at how you live at home. Earlier in the chapter, we covered the impact that screens can have on us versus natural light, and we just discussed the importance of changing visual attention for more positive mood shifts when looking at screens for prolonged periods. We will cover day–night rhythms and how they can be impacted by artificial light in more detail in the chapter on sleep from page 253. But there are other aspects of being indoors that you might not realise could be impacting your health.

The World Health Organization considers pollution *indoors*, as well as outdoors, a contributor to poor health.[90] This is most commonly from indoor smoke generated by having open fires and from cooking with open flame. But there are many other indoor pollutants that are relevant for our health. Do you use air fresheners?

Perhaps you use plug-ins, hanging air fresheners for the car, synthetic fabric freshener sprays . . . I know I have. The use of these products releases VOCs (volatile organic compounds) into the air, which can react with the ozone to produce secondary pollutants such as formaldehyde, secondary organic aerosol (SOA) and ultrafine particles (UFP). Obvious health symptoms from high exposure can be eye, lung or skin irritation. But longer-term health effects could arise years later, impacting our hormone regulation, lungs, heart and central nervous system.[91]

What about cleaning products? We have been using bleach products as disinfectants for over 170 years, and although bleach is very useful, it has been established that bleach exposure in workplace environments can negatively affect our lungs.[92] Studies also show using bleach at home is associated with adult-onset asthma in women, and passive exposure seems to increase the risk of lung infections in children too.[93,94]

I like lighting a candle at home very much. It can help evoke a feeling of calm and low ambient light in the evening that helps me to unwind. But scented candles also emit small particles and gases that pollute indoor air.[95] Exposure to fine particles in outdoor air has been convincingly linked to cardiovascular and respiratory events, so although we don't have specific data on indoor air and candle use in this context it does follow that indoor exposure could impact those vulnerable to lung issues. A recent study points to headaches, shortness of breath and coughing being associated with scented candle use.[96]

I am also a fan of incense. It has been a part of religious and cultural practices for Christians, Jews, Muslims, Buddhists and Taoists for thousands of years. In countries where Buddhism and Taoism are mainstream, incense burning at home is a daily practice. But air pollution at home and in, and around, temples has been documented to have harmful effects on health.[97] Burning any sort of

organic material, whether tobacco leaves, coal or an incense stick –
produces polyaromatic hydrocarbons, which have also been linked
to cancer.[98,99]

So what can you do?

I enjoy incense and candles, and I use them at home myself.
But being aware of the long-term health aspects of these products
means you have choice in how you use them.

Tips for a healthy home

- ❀ **Regularly open windows and doors** for proper air circulation.

- ❀ **If you use scented candles or incense, keep the space well ventilated**. It's possible that pure beeswax and soy wax candles may burn 'cleaner', thereby emitting less soot, but there is not much research on this.

- ❀ **Instead of synthetic air fresheners, you can use a reed diffuser** or mist diffuser that uses essential oils in water.

- ❀ **Use bleach very sparingly** or replace with more eco-friendly, 'non-toxic' cleaning products.

- ❀ **Make your own cleaning products!** These are cheaper and can smell better too. A general all-purpose cleaner in a spray bottle can be made with white vinegar and water in equal amounts, with lemon rind and rosemary sprigs as an optional addition. For kitchen cleaning, baking soda can deodorise and shine stainless steel; just combine baking soda and water to make a paste and rub surfaces with a damp cloth.

- ❀ **Consider investing in a HEPA air purifier** – the most effective way to clean the air, but also expensive.

Houseplants

If you can't get out in nature, be sure to bring nature into your home. The famous 1989 NASA Clean Air study found that indoor plants could remove compounds like benzene, formaldehyde and ammonia from the air. It identified seven top air-purifying plants: weeping fig, devil's ivy, Chinese evergreen, flamingo lily, bamboo palm, peace lily and fern.[100] Don't get too excited, though – although plants can reduce volatile organic compounds (VOCs) in small, sealed chambers, in a living space of 1,500 square feet, you'd need 680 houseplants to purify the air![101]

Luckily, houseplants have many other benefits: one study reported that when young adults touched houseplant foliage or smelled their blossoms, they noticed a reduction in both mental stress and physical signs of bodily stress.[102] It's also been shown that keeping plants around can make you physically healthier in all sorts of ways. Studies have noted improvements in the brain's electrical activity, lowered muscle tension, and improved blood pressure and healthier heart activity (heart rate variability).[103] Many of the benefits of plants at home can also be translated to the workplace. One study showed 'green' offices containing plants make staff happier and increase productivity by 15 per cent.[104] The research showed plants in the office significantly increased workplace satisfaction, concentration, and perceived air quality. There is some truth to this; although plants don't clean VOCs from the air in the average room, they will clean up some of the mould, bacteria, mildew or dust in their surroundings. In rooms that held plants, researchers found 50 to 60 per cent fewer bacteria and spores of mould than in rooms that lacked plant life.[105] I love my houseplants and take great pleasure in watering them. Seeing them grow and knowing they are helping us have clean air in our house brings me genuine joy each morning. It's so easy and provides you with the therapeutic benefits of being close to nature without having to change your lifestyle in a big way.

Homewares, plastics, cosmetics and personal-care products

I want to include a brief note here about other factors in our homes that can impact our health. We are surrounded by a number of different chemicals in our day-to-day lives that we don't tend to think about. In truth, research has never been done into the potential effects on the human body of these environmental chemicals in combination. You may have seen kids' plastic bottles labelled 'BPA-free' and wondered what it meant.[106,107] You may have seen that Teflon-coated pans had to stop using a chemical called PFOA since 2013.[108,109] These measures were taken because of the health risks associated with exposure to these substances. But health risks do not only come from one component of plastics or one chemical used in industrial processes. Legislation is slow to catch up, and many of these substances have yet to be investigated in combination. We not only drink from, or cook with, substances that have been associated with potential health risks. We also apply them to our skin (in creams, washes, gels, shampoos, make-ups and perfumes),[110,111] nails (in nail glue, acrylic and varnish removers)[112] and inside our bodies (personal-care products, tampons and pads).[113] They are everywhere.

I want to take a hopeful tone when it comes to understanding some of these exposures, though. For most of us, the majority of these products will have no noticeable health impacts. But it is worth being aware of them, as some of us may be more sensitive to the effects of prolonged exposures to these chemicals from multiple sources.

Let's take plastics as an example.

Recent evidence indicates that humans constantly inhale and ingest microplastics,[114] from obvious sources such as bottled water, Tupperware and cellophane-wrapped food, to the less obvious such as blends of synthetic, plastic-based fibres (polyester, nylon and polyamine) that can shed from our clothes (in wearing and washing them) and are also contained in non-cotton bed linen, carpets and soft toys. Even my favourite beverage, the humble cup of tea, can be affected. Many brands of paper tea bag use plastic sealants, and often the posh, silken, pyramid tea bags are made from polyethylene terephthalate (PET) or nylon (some are made from corn starch, which is ideal, so it is worth checking the brand). Research reveals that when you steep just one of these tea bags in hot water to make your tea, it breaks down to release over 11 billion microplastic particles *and over* 3 billion nanoplastics into your mug.[115] Somewhat off-putting.

This is pretty scary stuff. But does the science show there is actually something to worry about? Well, yes. It has been fairly well established that components of plastics (BPA, BPS, phthalates) and other chemicals in our environment (such as dioxins, PCBs and pesticides) can be so-called 'endocrine disruptors', which means they can impact how our bodies make and regulate hormones.[116,117] Windows of exposure (in pregnancy, and as a baby in the womb) can be important, as well as long-term exposures. We need more research to fully understand the potential impacts on us in terms of fertility, cancer risks and hormonal disorders from significant exposures to these substances.[118-121]

What can we do? Well, we know that stress can also impact health, so try not to ruminate on what you cannot change. If we are aware of limiting our long-term exposures to some of these substances, in ways that feel manageable and affordable, then I believe that is a good thing.

I have compiled a list of possible ideas that could help you reduce your 'substance burden'. It is not exhaustive. And you do not need to do everything here! They are just practical suggestions that could help you feel empowered and healthy in the modern world.

Tips for reducing plastic and chemical exposures at home

- **Try to keep plastic items out of direct sunlight** as this causes materials to break down and release airborne microplastics.
- **Drink tap water over bottled water** if you have a choice, as it tends to contain fewer microplastics.[122]
- **Drink loose-leaf tea with a strainer,** or use organic, paper- or corn starch-based tea bags.
- **If you can, use glass, ceramic or stainless-steel** Tupperware to store food.
- **Take your own metal or ceramic reusable cup to coffee shops** – or order your tea and coffee to drink in the shop. Paper cups that are designed to keep your drink warm contain a polyethylene layer.
- **Warm your food on the hob**, or in glass or ceramic crockery in the microwave.
- **If you have Teflon-coated pans, make sure you have some food or liquid in them before you apply heat.** Empty pans preheated can reach high temperatures, potentially releasing polymer fumes.
- **Ventilate your kitchen.** When you're cooking, turn on your extractor fan, or open a window to help clear any fumes.
- **Avoid using steel wool or scouring pads on nonstick pans,** since they can scratch the surface. Use wooden,

silicone or plastic utensils instead. Gently wash pots and pans with a sponge and soapy, warm water.

- ✸ **Replace old cookware.** When Teflon coatings start to scratch, peel, flake or chip, they are ready to be replaced. If you're buying new cooking pans, consider stainless steel, ceramic or cast iron.
- ✸ **When replacing furniture, carpets or toys, you can be mindful of using natural materials** that don't contain plastic, where possible.
- ✸ **Plastics like PCBs and dioxins tend to accumulate most in animal-based foods,** so consider a more plant-rich diet to limit these exposures (see the next chapter).
- ✸ **Wash your hands with normal soap** – there's no need for antibacterial soap. Good handwashing and drying reduces infection risk, regardless of whether soap contains antibacterial properties.
- ✸ **When they need replacing, consider looking for eco-friendly cosmetics** and personal-care products; they tend to be better for the environment and your body.
- ✸ **Spray perfumes on your clothes** more than on your skin.
- ✸ **If you are ever looking to invest in a water filter,** you can look for a non-plastic stainless-steel filter or a reverse osmosis water filter.

That list may have felt overwhelming. I know when I began to understand some of these potential areas I wanted to change, it felt like too much. But remember, you don't have to be perfect or become a zero-waste eco-warrior to make a few free and easy changes to your lifestyle. Just take it slowly and see what fits into your life. When the time comes for making a bigger purchase, e.g. a new cookware item, you'll simply be aware of the kind of thing to look for.

Let me share a story with you. A 30-year-old woman came to see me with Hashimoto's thyroiditis, which is a type of thyroid problem caused by an autoimmune process in the body. I'll call her Rachel. She was experiencing low energy, dry skin and weight gain, and she had also been feeling low in mood over the preceding months. Once diagnosed, Rachel received thyroid hormone replacement, which really helped her symptoms. But we also looked at ways her diet and her environment could be changed, with the hope of reducing the thyroid-specific antibodies (TPO antibodies) her body was making, and generally improve her well-being. We focused on an anti-inflammatory diet rich in fibre, with the right amount of iodine, selenium, iron and healthy fatty acids.[123] But we also looked at making sure she had the right levels of vitamin D, a good sleep and movement routine, and lastly, we looked at her environment as well. For Rachel, this was the hardest part. She loved scented candles and was also fastidious when it came to cleaning her home. She used a lot of cleaning products with chemicals, as well as regular trips to the nail salon for acrylic nails. She also regularly used air fresheners, tanning sprays and perfumes and had never thought about her exposure to plastics before. She found that results from her new diet happened quickly, and it led to some great reductions in her TPO antibodies. She felt better on more sleep and with regular outdoor walks too. But, interestingly, her TPO antibodies went down the most after she began looking at her home environment.

Over the course of several months, she began to implement some of the tips I mentioned above. She started using glass Tupperware, eco-friendly cleaning products, personal-care products and make-up. She invested in a HEPA air filter. She became passionate about eco-friendly cleansers, body washes and creams too. Whether it was several months of diet and lifestyle changes, the shifts she had made in her home environment, or perhaps all of these things is hard to say. But, amazingly, her TPO antibody levels normalised, and she was even able to reduce her thyroid hormone replacement significantly too. I'd love to see more research in the coming years looking at the cumulative impacts of multiple chemical exposures. But until then, a simple rule of thumb is that what's good for the planet is probably good for you too.

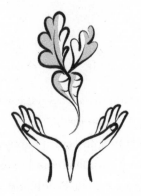

Vegetables

Did your grandma always tell you to 'eat your veggies'? There's a reason for that sage advice. Vegetables are one of the most underrated parts of a happy and healthy lifestyle. Plants – vegetables, fruits, wholegrains, beans, peas, herbs, spices, nuts and seeds – are vital for our health and, in general, few of us eat enough.

There is a huge body of research that shows how heart disease, cancer, and hormone, skin and gut health are all impacted by our food choices. It was an accumulation of years of research and a labour of love for me to write my first book, which focused on this evidence.[1] For many people, changing their eating habits might seem like the easiest first step towards improved health, while perhaps changing your home environment or working on your emotional health with gratitude and love exercises might seem like a greater stretch. I go into the science of a wholefoods, plant-based diet in my first book, *The Plant Power Doctor*. In this chapter, I will summarise the science in a more succinct way, and I've got some new delicious recipes from some good friends of mine, to help you eat more veg!

Why do I recommend a plant-based diet? What is interesting to know is that although a plant-rich diet can look different for various cultures, the research is remarkably consistent in promoting the power of plants.[2-10] This is especially true when you take a step back and look at large populations of people, and how they build healthy habits. Incredibly, just four health conditions account for *80 per cent* of all premature deaths globally: heart disease, cancers, lung disease and diabetes.[11] And the crazy part? About

80 per cent of these premature deaths could be prevented by adopting four healthy lifestyle factors:

❀ a healthy diet predominantly consisting of plants
❀ regular physical activity
❀ not smoking
❀ a sensible use of alcohol.[12]

Does this surprise you? As a doctor, I spend most of my day helping people when they are *already affected* by these conditions. How wonderful it is to be able to share this information with you *before* you begin to live with a life-limiting disease.

Is there one of these healthy habits that has the highest impact? Yes, it is our diet.

Globally, it is reported that unhealthy diets contribute to more death and disability than smoking, alcohol and drug use combined.[13] Wow. The most comprehensive analysis of risk factors has determined that one in five deaths are caused by an unhealthy diet.[14]

Diets low in wholegrains, fruit, nuts, seeds and vegetables, and high in salt and saturated fat (mainly from eating meat and ultra-processed foods), are the least healthy.[15]

Research has shown us that there are also a number of specific health concerns that can also be improved through a daily habit of eating more plants. We can:

❀ Reduce the risk of developing the vast majority of heart disease.[2,8,9]
❀ Reduce the risk of developing certain cancers and help us recover from cancer treatments and their side effects.[16-23]
❀ Prevent us from developing type 2 diabetes and help us reverse it if we do have it.[10,26,36]

- ❀ Maintain a healthy gut, reduce the risk of diverticular disease and inflammatory bowel disease.[24,25,37]
- ❀ Improve our hormone regulation.[5,36,38]
- ❀ Reduce period pains, fibroids and endometriosis as well as polycystic ovary syndrome (PCOS) and menopausal symptoms.[27,32-35]
- ❀ Improve skin health, acne, psoriasis and eczema.[41-43]
- ❀ Support immunity.[4,44-46]
- ❀ Help alleviate the symptoms of rheumatoid arthritis, lupus and multiple sclerosis.[28-31, 39, 40]

It may seem too good to be true, and certainly a healthy plant-focused diet is not a panacea. Many of us will still experience chronic disease, and of course, none of us lives forever. But I have nonetheless seen some incredible transformations in my own family and in the lives of my patients that are hard to ignore. Often, these patients also found unintended side effects from their lifestyle changes.

- ❀ One woman was hoping to improve her asthma, but found that her chronic kidney disease and liver disorder also improved.
- ❀ One man hoping to improve his chronic pain found his low-grade prostate cancer reversed.
- ❀ One woman who was hoping to improve her menopausal symptoms noticed a dramatic improvement to her mood and her lupus.

You don't need to immediately go on a fully plant-based diet (and it's important you are aware that a lot of vegan ready-made food is not healthy and is ultra-processed too). I also really would not want you to read this and feel anxious about what you eat.

Putting too much pressure on yourself and feeling restricted is not a sustainable way to create habits. You must decide what you feel you can include and maintain in your life, rather than a 'quick fix'. But by increasing your intake of plant-based wholefoods, the evidence shows you can only do good for your long-term health. It's not so much about the occasional food choice that we make, but more the *dietary pattern* that we follow as a whole, which has the biggest impact on our health. A pain au chocolat with friends may be the perfect food/social activity pairing to boost your mood! It is important to be aware that maintaining a healthy lifestyle means choosing fatty, sweet and salty foods less often than we choose plant-based wholefoods.

My husband decided he wanted to adopt a fully plant-based diet before I did, and I remember asking him how he could stick with it for every meal. He used to eat so much cheese! I wasn't sure if I could do it. He replied that for him, making the decision was easy, because it was not only for his own health, but it became something more important to him. He felt it was consistent with his values of protecting the environment and of animal welfare. It therefore became a part of who he felt he was.

Not everyone feels this way. I certainly didn't at first. But I could clearly see that for him, a shift in identity became important in helping him stick with it. It made the changes easier than will-power ever could, which research shows us doesn't last.

The best way to achieve a healthier life is through simple shifts towards healthful choices that you can keep doing – things that feel enjoyable. By adding in more of the foods that will nourish and sustain you, and crowding out the ones that don't. Little shifts like making your morning cuppa and taking it outside for some fresh air and daylight before you start your day. Maybe doing some jumping jacks or squats while you wait for your kettle to boil. By choosing small steps you can easily do, habits turn into patterns and patterns turn into a healthy life.

Eating for the planet

Plant-based diets do not just benefit us. As David Attenborough so eloquently pointed out in the BBC documentary *A Life on Our Planet*, by eating a plant-based diet we are doing the single biggest thing any individual can do to help mitigate climate change.

According to the UN, the animal-agriculture industry contributes not only to climate change, but also to infectious diseases, water pollution, land degradation, species extinction and air pollution.[47] We breed roughly 70 billion land animals to kill and eat each year. To feed these 70 billion animals, we need large amounts of crops that destroy ecosystems, and we use nitrogen fertilisers, which seep into the oceans. This causes algal blooms, acidifying the water and causing dead zones. We must give the animals antibiotics when they get sick from overcrowding. In some countries, approximately 80 per cent of overall antibiotic use is in the animal sector.[48] Overuse and misuse of antibiotics in animals is contributing to the rising threat of antibiotic resistance in humans; a UN Report tells us antibiotic resistant infections could cause 10 million human deaths each year by 2050.[49] Shockingly, by 2030, antimicrobial resistance could force up to 24 million people into extreme poverty.[50]

Eating fish also contributes to the planet's problems; surprisingly, fishing boats that trawl the ocean floor release as much carbon dioxide as the entire aviation industry.[51] Meanwhile, commercial fishing gear is one of the most common ocean plastics. In the North Highlands of Scotland, discarded fishing gear makes up 90 per cent of ocean plastic removed by beach cleaners.[52] Fishing lines, ropes and nets make up around half of the plastic pollution in the Great Pacific Garbage Patch.[53] Sadly, microplastics could also affect human health; studies show they are absorbed through the air we breathe, the food we eat, the water we drink and even through our skin.[54] Although more research is needed on the impact this has on our health, we know that microplastics can have effects on human hormones and placenta function.[55,56] It seems that whatever we do to the planet and its creatures, we also ultimately do to ourselves.

Eating for the future

A 2021 report published by UNICEF found that one billion children are at 'extreme risk' from the impact of climate change – things like coastal flooding, infectious diseases, heatwaves, and water scarcity are some of the reasons why.[57] Species are becoming extinct 100 times faster than they would without animal agriculture. Populations of wild animals have more than halved since 1970, while the human population has doubled. Only five times before in our planet's history have so many species been lost so quickly; the fifth time was when the dinosaurs were wiped out. That is why scientists and conservationists call what is happening now the 'sixth mass extinction'. This era, of human impact on the planet, has officially been dubbed 'the Anthropocene'.[58]

I know this feels like a lot of doom and gloom, but I promise you *there is hope.*

The landmark 2019 EAT-*Lancet* Commission report on feeding the world sustainably concluded that, with radical changes to food production and consumption, providing enough nutrition for everyone is possible.[59] But in order to do it, we have to eat more plants. Thankfully, a healthy, plant-based diet is a sustainable way of eating, which can future-proof our own health and that of the planet for the next generation. But how can we *connect* to this information, to help us really care enough to change our own habits day to day?

I hope, as you read, you can see how gratitude (G), love (L), going outside (O), and eating vegetables (V) is all connected – because our health is linked to the health of everyone around us, and the world around us too.

By nourishing our bodies we can help prevent diseases, but another way in which our nutrition can encourage life-long positive changes is through how we actually *feel*.

Mood food

There are many ways you can help to boost your mood, including getting enough sleep and exercise, and having positive social bonds, as we explore elsewhere in this book. If you are struggling, please remember that mental illness is complicated. If you feel suicidal or have been diagnosed with bipolar disorder, I will never tell you to eat more broccoli or get a hobby. If you are living with trauma and PTSD, no amount of healthy food and exercise changes will 'fix' what you are having to live with.

Some of us will suffer from mental health issues despite adopting all or many lifestyle changes into our routines – because human emotions and experiences are often far more complicated and nuanced than what I can cover in this book. Please do not suffer alone. What I hope is that this section offers you some new things to try that could help you, and help you consider your diet and how it might be impacting your body. Try the ideas here alongside the self-care suggestions for mental and emotional well-being throughout this book, as well as medicine if needed, and therapy.

Can we really eat for a healthy mind?

I had a patient a few years back who was struggling with peri-menopause. She decided to make some diet changes to see if it would help her hot flushes. When she came back to me a few months later, her flushes having resolved, she had also experienced other unexpected benefits. Better sleep, weight loss and friends had even told her she looked younger! But one of the things she was not expecting was how good she was feeling mentally. Her anxiety had lifted, and she admitted that for her, a shift in her mood was a lovely added benefit of a wholefoods, plant-based diet. It was the main reason she felt so excited with the diet changes she had made.

Is this something that's been observed in the scientific litera-ture? Have any studies looking at real people over time shown the food and mood link to be true? It turns out that yes, there are some potential links with food and mood. A meta-analysis (which is generally the most reliable form of study) published in *Psychosomatic Medicine* looked at nearly 46,000 people, and it con-cluded that diet changes can significantly improve anxiety. Researchers reviewed 16 studies that reported effects of healthful dietary interventions on depression and anxiety. Diets that reduced the intake of fatty foods, such as processed meats, led to signifi-cantly decreased symptoms of depression, compared with control diets. Increased intake of fibre, minerals, and vitamins from fruits and vegetables may improve pathways related to depression, including inflammation and oxidative stress.[60]

There have also been interesting trials using food as an active treatment for depression. In the 'SMILES' trial, half the partici-pants were supported in adopting a Mediterranean-style diet and the other half were in a social-support control group. Those in the first group had significant improvements to their mental health, with 32 per cent of these participants reporting resolution of symptoms after 12 weeks compared to 8 per cent of the social-support group.[61] In another trial they reported using a wholefoods, plant-based lunchtime intervention programme at an insurance company over several sites. They offered a once weekly education session plus the opportunity to eat a healthy vegan meal each lunchtime should they wish to. The study involved nearly 300 people who were overweight or who had type 2 diabetes. Not only did the participants improve their cardiac risk factors during the time of the study, they also noted improvements in rates of depression and anxiety among the participants, as well as improved productivity in the workplace.[62]

Let's look at how your emotions, mind and body are connected and influenced by what you eat and how you can get more of these crucial nutrients into your daily diet.

The food we eat is really information. Food molecules break down and interact with our hormones, our immune system and our digestive system and are ultimately incorporated into our DNA.

It's actually possible to detect microRNA (miRNA), a class of non-coding RNAs that play important roles in regulating gene expression, in our bodies from some of the foods we ingest. For example, miRNA from cow's milk that we drink, and the meat and even the crops we eat (including rice), have been detected circulating in our bloodstream – taking the term 'you are what you eat' literally.[63] I love to imagine the food we eat breaking down into molecules that flow to all the cells in our bodies, almost like music reverberating through our blood, lymphatics and nervous system to improve our health.

Food impacts our mood once it is in our digestive system. The gut is truly incredible; referred to as the 'second brain', it is the only organ to have its own independent nervous system, an intricate network of 100 million neurons embedded in the gut wall. There are three main ways this nutritional information interacts with our gut to affect our mood: through the vagus nerve, the lymphatic system and the microbiome.

The vagus nerve conveys information from the base of the brain – the medulla oblongata – to the gut and back again. In fact, the signals from the gut to the brain through the vagus nerve out-number the brain instructions to the gut by about ten to one – our gut talks to our brain much more than our brain talks to our gut! I think of visceral feelings, 'gut instincts', as emotional messages transferred up to your brain via the vagus nerve.

Eighty per cent of the immune cells in our bodies reside in the gut, which provides a rich communication between our lymphatic system (the fluid in our bodies that transports immune cells) and our microbes (bacteria, viruses and others that reside outside the gut walls).[64] These relationships are complex, but studies do show our moods can be affected by the amount of white blood cells (which fight infection) that are in our bloodstream.[65] The cells of our immune system can also attach to our hormones (that can then affect our mood), such as thyroid hormones, oestrogen and testosterone.[66-68]

The third important way our food communicates with our brain is via gut bugs. Your microbiome, made up of a range of microbes, communicates with your gut and immune system too. The micro-biome contributes to inflammation in the gut – both the prevention of it and its creation, depending on which bacteria are present and how strong the gut-wall function is.[69] Lots of emerging evidence now also points to the role that inflammation in the body has in affecting our moods.[70,71] How does the gut wall affect inflammation? The gut lining is only one cell thick, and the immune cells living right next to it are our first line of defence against potential pathogens in our gut, absorbed from the outside world, from getting inside our bodies. When the gut lining is damaged, those bugs seep through the weakened gut lining and into our bodies.[72] This is called intestinal permeability. When we eat foods with saturated fat in the diet (from meat, cheese and junk foods), this is one of the ways in which the gut can become 'leaky' and lead to endotoxaemia, a phenomenon where bacteria cross the gut barrier to end up in the bloodstream.[73,74] Our immune cells then react to this and inflammation occurs. This process potentially increases our risk of a number of mental, physical and emotional conditions, from rheumatoid arthritis to Alzheimer's.[75-77]

The good news is that one of the ways that our gut lining can be protected is by eating more fibre.[78] Amazingly, when we eat fibre, it is the perfect fuel for beneficial gut bugs. They ferment the fibre to create metabolites called short-chain fatty acids (SCFAs), which are great for our health.[79] They have a 'soothing effect' on the body, strengthening the gut lining, reducing inflammation, improving metabolism and even reducing the risk of certain cancers.[80] And in the context of mood, they may also reduce symptoms of depression and irritable bowel syndrome.[81] How? The brain has a special protective barrier (the aptly named 'blood–brain barrier') inside the blood vessels supplying the central nervous system. This barrier tightly regulates the movement of ions, molecules and cells between the blood and the brain. SCFAs are able to cross this barrier and get into the brain, reducing inflammation in our brain cells.[82] Amazingly, SCFAs also have a role in strengthening the blood–brain barrier, thereby protecting the brain.[83]

'Psychobiotics'

The brain also affects our gut-bug populations – studies have shown that psychological stress suppresses beneficial bacteria. In one study, researchers found that during exam week, university students' stool samples contained fewer lactobacilli, a key 'good' bacterium that serves as a probiotic, than they had during the stress-free first days of the semester.[84] Major shifts in gut-bug populations have been observed not just in depression and anxiety, but also for more complex diagnoses affecting our brains, such as dementia.[85] The science into how bacteria can influence our mood is a burgeoning area of research, and researchers have given the microbiota that affect our wellbeing the catchy name of 'psychobiotics'.

Good-mood food

We still have much to learn. Until we know more, the key message is: eat more fibre to feed the bacteria in your gut that protect your gut lining. This encourages a positive conversation between your gut, brain and immune system.

There are other components in food that could also boost your mood:

- ❀ **Vitamin B12, folate and vitamin B6.** These three vitamins help to break down an amino acid associated with low mood and dementia – homocysteine.[86] A fruit- and vegetable-rich plate is abundant in B6 and folate, and they can also be found in wholegrains, beans, lentils, nuts and seeds. For vitamin B12, it is crucial to supplement or eat fortified foods (plant milks, cereals, Marmite, nutritional yeast) if you are on a fully plant-based diet. B12 supplementation is also important for anyone (including meat-eaters) over the age of 50, or those unable to absorb vitamin B12 well (people with reflux, coeliac disease or digestion issues, for example), so as to ensure homocysteine is broken down effectively.

❋ **Folate**, found mainly from green leafy vegetables, may also play a role in helping mood in other ways.[87] A prospective follow-up study showed low dietary folate increases risk for severe depression by as much as threefold.[88] But the same benefits for mood are not found with folate supplements – it has to be the real deal, fruits and vegetables, to make a difference.

❋ **Carotenoids** (from yellow- and orange-coloured fruits and veggies). One survey showed the participants' mood scores lifted exactly in line with the amount of carotenoid-rich foods they were eating.[89] It seems the natural antioxidants contained in fruits and vegetables alongside the folate may be crucial in reaping the benefits for our mood and health.

We also know a few things that work to bring our mood down, and so should be minimised wherever possible:

❋ **Artificial sweeteners and sugar-sweetened drinks** are associated with increased risk of irritability and depression in some small studies.[90] Aspartame, which is present in thousands of products, including mints, gum, cereals and snack bars, has been shown to be harmful to our gut microbiota, and one human study noted it had an effect on vulnerable populations already suffering from mental health problems.[91] The International Agency for Research on Cancer put aspartame into the category of possibly carcinogenic (but the evidence was of a similar strength to things like mobile phone use and pickled vegetables, so it is by no means conclusive). More data are needed in humans to draw conclusions, and for most people, having sensible amounts of artificial sweeteners in their diet will be fine. Maybe your weekly Diet Coke brings a source of joy to your life! It is also important to recognise artificial sweeteners are a useful tool for limiting sugar in fizzy drinks for people with weight-loss goals. But remember, reducing our exposure to these hyper-sweet flavours could also help our taste buds to favour wholefoods and fruits over time.

❀ **Caffeine.** Given how much we know about caffeine and its disruption of normal sleep patterns, I'd recommend enjoying no more than one or two cups of coffee a day – before midday if possible. Coffee has been shown to have some great health benefits, but caffeine can also increase levels of both cortisol and adrenaline, our main stress hormones. This will affect some of us more than others. If you are prone to anxiety and notice the effects of caffeine, this could be an obvious thing to cut back on.

A wholefoods, plant-powered diet

A plant-forward approach is all about understanding some of the rich variety and delicious ingredients of a plant-powered menu.

I want you to be familiar with the kinds of foods that contain vital nutrients that give us energy and plant power, which can be incorporated into any culture or cuisine. That way, it will be easier for you to remember to add variety to your meal plans to ensure maximum flavour and nutrition.

I go into lots of detail on this in my first book, *The Plant Power Doctor*. Another good place to start is the *Plant-Based Eatwell Guide*, which was formulated by dieticians, doctors and nutrition researchers to emulate the UK's 2016 healthy-eating manual, the *Eatwell Guide*, but with the exclusion of animal products. It gives a good foundation of information to understand how to achieve a sustainable and healthy diet with different food groups, shown in the proportions that they should contribute to your overall diet.

The 2019 Canadian Dietary Guidelines are also a useful reference. They emphasise plant proteins and encourage plenty of vegetables and fruit, water and wholegrain foods and exclude dairy as a necessary food group. I'm a fan of how this guideline encourages a more mindful approach, as well as suggesting we prioritise eating with others, cook at home more often and check nutrition labels on ready-made foods. What makes these recent dietary guidelines particularly useful is they were not influenced by industry agendas (which can sometimes happen when agricultural activity and economic influences are taken into account).

Let's go through a quick summary of the most important nutrients to focus on in a plant-based diet and where they are found.

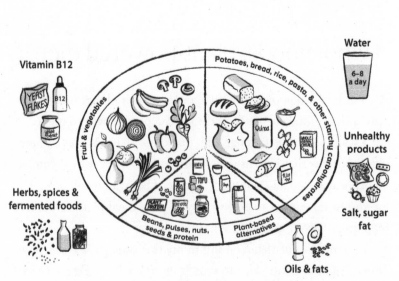

The Plant-Based Eatwell Guide.

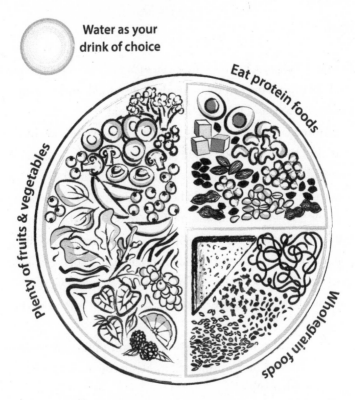

The 2019 Canadian Dietary Guidelines.

This will boost your confidence when thinking about what foods you enjoy, and the meals you want to make with them at home.

Nutrients to focus on

Protein

Beans, lentils, chickpeas, tofu, soy alternatives to milk and yoghurt, peanuts and nut butter. Other ideas include cashew nuts, pistachios, chia seeds, ground flaxseed, pumpkin seeds, buckwheat, quinoa and wild rice.

Iron

Lentils, chickpeas, beans, tofu, cashew nuts, chia seeds, ground linseed, hemp seeds, pumpkin seeds, kale, dried apricots and figs, raisins, quinoa and fortified breakfast cereal.

More plant-sourced iron is absorbed when your body is short of iron, and less is absorbed when your stores are full. Tea, coffee and some substances in plant foods may make it difficult for your body to absorb iron. So a top tip would be to avoid tea and coffee with meals.

The good news is that vitamin C increases iron absorption. Good sources of vitamin C include peppers (yellow and red especially), broccoli, cabbage, Brussels sprouts, kiwis, oranges, strawberries, pineapple, grapefruit and orange juice. Combine iron-rich and vitamin-C-rich ingredients in your meals to maximise absorption! Some ideas include:

* porridge made with water or plant milk, with ground flaxseed and raisins, eaten alongside a small glass of orange juice
* a lentil curry followed by a kiwi
* a tofu stir-fry with broccoli or a bean chilli with red pepper.

Iodine

The amount of iodine in a plant food varies depending on how much iodine was in the soil the plant was grown in. Although seaweed is a rich source, the iodine content varies, and is sometimes too high. Iodised salt is a traditional source, but if we want to cut down on salt, another option is to use a plant milk fortified with iodine – look for potassium iodide in the ingredients list. I think a non-seaweed iodine supplement is the most reliable way of meeting your body's need for iodine. Along with iodine, selenium is also important for thyroid hormone production. It is often available in supplement form, or one or two Brazil nuts a day will easily cover your selenium needs.

Calcium

Calcium-set tofu, broccoli, cauliflower, watercress, Brussels sprouts, kale, pak choi, okra, spring greens, dried figs, chia seeds, almonds, almond butter, calcium-fortified milk and yoghurt alternatives and bread fortified with calcium.

Vitamin D

Whatever our diet, supplementation with vitamin D is an important consideration – see page 106.

Vitamin B12

Vitamin B12 is made by microorganisms, and isn't produced by plants, so I'd recommend taking a supplement. Take 10mcg (micrograms) daily or 2000mcg weekly. Your body absorbs vitamin B12 more efficiently in frequent, small amounts, so the less often you have it, the more you need. You may notice that there are supplements containing different types of vitamin B12. Cyanocobalamin is recommended, mainly because it is the most stable type. Your body converts it to the two active forms of vitamin B12. Many foods are now fortified with B12 too, if you'd rather meet your needs that way. Vitamin B12 is added to some plant milks, margarines, yeast extracts like Marmite, and breakfast cereals. Nutritional yeast flakes (or 'nooch') also contain Vitamin B12; you can try these on popcorn or sprinkled on pasta, stews or salads. Nooch also helps to make cheesy sauces delicious. If you rely only on fortified foods, you'll need to aim to eat these foods at least twice a day for a daily intake of 3mcg.

Zinc

Beans, chickpeas, lentils, tofu, tempeh, miso, walnuts, cashew nuts, chia seeds, ground flaxseed, hemp seeds, pumpkin seeds, wholemeal bread and quinoa.

Omega-3s

A tablespoon of ground flaxseed daily is a great source of short-chain omega-3s. I'd suggest you sprinkle it into porridge, stews, curries, yoghurts or whatever you usually eat. For long-chain omega-3s, we can supplement with EPA and DHA from microalgae too, which may be particularly important for infants and those who are pregnant or breastfeeding, but more research is needed. To understand more about healthy fats, see the next section on healthy fats.

Healthy fats

Plant-based diets should include healthy fats. Monounsaturated fatty acids (MUFAs) are often in nuts, and polyunsaturated fatty acids (PUFAs) are often in seeds – both of which are important components of a healthy diet. PUFAs include alpha-linolenic acid

(ALA), which makes omega-3s, and linoleic acid (LA), which makes omega-6 fatty acids.

Both are important but often omega-3s are harder to come by, so we should give them more attention when it comes to what we eat. Think of flaxseed, chia seeds, hemp seeds and walnuts as great sources of ALA.

Long-chain omega-3 fats (EPA and DHA) can be made in the body using the parent fat ALA, but this process can be inefficient and may happen less when there are other fats crowding out the conversion required. This is why sometimes ready-made long-chain omega-3s are useful. They can be found in fish, and for plant-based eaters, they can be found in algae (which is how the fish obtain it). This is where algae-oil supplements could be useful, but more data is needed to know for sure.

There are certainly many vegetarian populations that do not consume algae oil and have not experienced poor health outcomes as a result of avoiding fish.[92] So although omega-3s are healthful and necessary, the jury is still out on whether algae-oil supplements are a must-have. The important thing to remember is that in replacing saturated fats (primarily found in meat, cheese, eggs and junk food) with MUFAs and PUFAs we can improve cholesterol levels and reduce the risk of heart disease. Think of almonds, cashews, pecans, Brazil nuts, peanuts and avocados for MUFAs, and walnuts, sunflower seeds, flaxseed and peanuts for PUFAs.

When using oils, the best studies we have looking at large populations of people and what they eat actually show that replacing saturated fats in the diet (from sources such as meat or butter) with PUFA- and MUFA-rich oils such as rapeseed oil actually reduces cardiovascular disease risk.[93,94] Seed oils are not the enemy they have been made out to be. Extra virgin olive oil is associated with health benefits, but like any oil, it is calorie dense – so if weight loss is your aim, use small amounts.

For some people, oils can seem to trigger autoimmune flare-ups, e.g. inflammatory arthritis, though we have no studies to show this. Plant-based, no-oil diets have also been used to improve symptoms associated with heart disease.[95] If this is a concern for you, no-oil cooking is a convenient way to minimise oils in the diet.

Tips for no-oil cooking

- ❀ **High heat on your pan** will allow your veg to brown, which will add extra flavour when cooking without oil.
- ❀ **Deglaze.** When using onions or garlic, sauté them with a dash of water and herbs and spices, allowing them to absorb the flavours. Then keep adding a tablespoon or so of water or veg stock to deglaze the pan (scrape the browning with a wooden or silicone spatula) and get the most out of the developing flavours.
- ❀ **Get creative!** You can add some low-salt tamari for a salty, rich flavour or some balsamic vinegar for a sweeter, punchy flavour, cooking with onions or other vegetables for three to five minutes to allow for the tamari or vinegar to thicken.

For maximum health impact, you need a varied diet

This is a tried-and-true statement but perhaps not something people consider enough when eating a plants-only diet. Every plant has a unique mixture of antioxidants, polyphenols, vitamins and minerals which, when combined, provide powerful nutrients to nurture a range of beneficial gut microbes that are healthy for us. As much as I love carrots and peas, if I were to only eat carrots and peas, my gut would be missing out on important combinations of gut bugs that work together to create a cohesive ecosystem. This means eating as many different kinds of fruit, vegetables, wholegrains, beans, seeds, nuts, herbs and spices as we can.

You may have heard the phrase 'eat the rainbow'. This is why: different-coloured plant foods are more likely to contain different polyphenols that benefit us in synergistic ways.

In 2018, The American Gut Project, in collaboration with the University of California, released the findings of a huge survey they conducted of the microbiome of over 11,000 participants from 42 countries. One conclusion drawn was that the diversity of plants in our diet was the most powerful predictor of a healthy gut microbiome. Those who ate more than 30 different types of plants a week had the healthiest guts! That sounds like a lot, but I promise you it is easier than you think when you know how. It can help to think of 30 different plants in terms of 'plant points' that you can add up each week to get to 30. What counts as plant points? Any size serving of different types of vegetables, fruits, wholegrains, pulses and legumes, nuts and seeds all count as one point each. Different colours of the same vegetable or fruit count as distinct plants, e.g. if you eat a yellow and a red pepper, you've eaten two of your 30 plants for that week. Fresh, dried, canned and frozen plants also all count. Herbs and spices, extra virgin olive oil, tea and coffee are quarter of a point each.

All you have to do is get counting! Add up how many points are in each meal and snack, and over the course of a week if you manage 30+ plant points you are a plant point pro! Some families keep a chart in their kitchen, or compete with each other to get more plant points. Check out the table below if you want a tool to help you tick off your plant points. It can be printed and put on your fridge to make it even easier to be a plant point pro.

The plant points calculator

Here is a list to inspire you – can you tick off 30 plants over the course of the next week?

VEG (fresh or frozen)	1	2	3	4	5	6	7
Cruciferous vegetables (rocket, bok choy, broccoli, Brussels sprouts, cabbage, cauliflower, collard greens, horseradish, kale, radishes, watercress)	☐	☐	☐	☐	☐	☐	☐
Leafy greens (spinach, lettuce, spring greens)	☐	☐	☐	☐	☐	☐	☐
Salad (radishes, celery, cucumber, radicchio)	☐	☐	☐	☐	☐	☐	☐
Alliums (spring onions, onions, leeks, garlic)	☐	☐	☐	☐	☐	☐	☐
Root veg (carrots, beetroot, turnips, but not potatoes)	☐	☐	☐	☐	☐	☐	☐
Bell peppers, red chillies	☐	☐	☐	☐	☐	☐	☐
Peas	☐	☐	☐	☐	☐	☐	☐

	1	2	3	4	5	6	7
Mushrooms	☐	☐	☐	☐	☐	☐	☐
Tomatoes	☐	☐	☐	☐	☐	☐	☐
Avocados	☐	☐	☐	☐	☐	☐	☐
Aubergines, courgettes	☐	☐	☐	☐	☐	☐	☐
Corn, sweetcorn	☐	☐	☐	☐	☐	☐	☐
Asparagus, artichokes, celery	☐	☐	☐	☐	☐	☐	☐
Other	☐	☐	☐	☐	☐	☐	☐

FRUIT (fresh or frozen)

	1	2	3	4	5	6	7
Citrus fruit (lemons, oranges, grapefruit)	☐	☐	☐	☐	☐	☐	☐
Berries (blueberries, strawberries, raspberries, blackberries)	☐	☐	☐	☐	☐	☐	☐
Tree fruit (apples, pears, plums, peaches, nectarines, apricots, cherries, grapes)	☐	☐	☐	☐	☐	☐	☐
Bananas	☐	☐	☐	☐	☐	☐	☐
Kiwi, mangoes, pineapple, papaya, lychee, persimmons, custard apple, jackfruit	☐	☐	☐	☐	☐	☐	☐
Melons: honeydew, cantaloupe, Galia, watermelon	☐	☐	☐	☐	☐	☐	☐
Other	☐	☐	☐	☐	☐	☐	☐

WHOLEGRAINS	1	2	3	4	5	6	7
Rolled oats	☐	☐	☐	☐	☐	☐	☐
Rice (black, brown or wild rice are generally more nutritious than white)	☐	☐	☐	☐	☐	☐	☐
Oatcakes	☐	☐	☐	☐	☐	☐	☐
Gluten-free grains: quinoa, brown rice, corn, buckwheat, amaranth, polenta, sorghum, teff). Oats are also GF (if you have coeliac disease check the oats are certified 'gluten free')	☐	☐	☐	☐	☐	☐	☐
Wholewheat flour, bulgur wheat	☐	☐	☐	☐	☐	☐	☐
Wholegrain pasta	☐	☐	☐	☐	☐	☐	☐
Other	☐	☐	☐	☐	☐	☐	☐
PULSES AND LEGUMES (canned or cooked from dried)							
Chickpeas (including gram flour)	☐	☐	☐	☐	☐	☐	☐
Lentils (including lentil flour and lentil pasta)	☐	☐	☐	☐	☐	☐	☐
Beans (black, butter, cannellini, kidney, pinto, chickpeas, edamame, mung, yellow split peas)	☐	☐	☐	☐	☐	☐	☐
Other	☐	☐	☐	☐	☐	☐	☐

NUTS AND SEEDS
(not processed, unsalted)

	1	2	3	4	5	6	7
Almonds, walnuts, pecans, hazelnuts, cashews, peanuts, Brazil nuts, pistachios, macadamia, chestnut, pine nuts	☐	☐	☐	☐	☐	☐	☐
Other	☐	☐	☐	☐	☐	☐	☐

HERBS AND SPICES (fresh or dried)

	1	2	3	4	5	6	7
Cinnamon, cloves, nutmeg, star anise, ginger, cardamom	☐	☐	☐	☐	☐	☐	☐
Paprika, chilli powder/flakes, curry powder, cumin, mustard seeds, turmeric, garlic powder, black pepper	☐	☐	☐	☐	☐	☐	☐
Parsley, coriander, basil, oregano, sage, rosemary, mint	☐	☐	☐	☐	☐	☐	☐
Other	☐	☐	☐	☐	☐	☐	☐

Vegetables ....

Fruits ....

Wholegrains ....

Pulses and legumes ....

Nuts and seeds ....

Herbs and spices ....

TOTAL NO. ....

Tips for adding more plants to your meals

How did you do? If you came up a bit short, here are some quick ways to add more plants to your diet:

- ✿ Add mixed seeds to cereals or porridge.
- ✿ If cooking with mince, substitute half with lentils or beans, or use plant-based mince.
- ✿ Add flavour and texture to salads by adding some roasted chickpeas or nuts.
- ✿ Stir in a handful of spinach to stews or curries.
- ✿ Buy mixed packs of rice, berries, and frozen veg, and tins of mixed beans.
- ✿ Roast a big batch of various vegetables to keep in the fridge and use through the week.
- ✿ Subscribe to a veg box delivery service. This will help you to eat more seasonal vegetables and find new recipes to try.
- ✿ Add spelt or barley into stews or soups.
- ✿ Add an extra dried herb or spice to your meal. For instance, cumin tastes great mixed with turmeric, curry powder, cayenne, cinnamon, coriander, garlic, and saffron. It also pairs well with tomatoes and chickpeas.

Is mindful eating a health habit?

Mindful eating simply means taking time to eat, away from other distractions like your work screen, phone or TV. It's a way to appreciate your food and pay more attention to what you are putting into your body and how it makes you feel. It's important because it means you are slowing down your eating, chewing your food properly and allowing your mouth time to produce the salivary enzymes needed to break down your foods, as well as preparing your gut. It also allows you more opportunity to spot if a food is having a good or negative impact on your body – indigestion, wind, acid reflux, tummy ache, heartburn. Eating slowly helps your brain, salivary enzymes and gut prepare for the job at hand!

Tips for mindful eating

- ❀ **Sit at a table and put your food on a plate.** I often eat lunch at my desk from necessity, but I use a plate and take 15 minutes between calls and appointments if I can – without looking at my phone.
- ❀ **Set your fork down while you chew.** Can you manage more than ten chews each bite? How does it feel to chew more?
- ❀ **Eat your last meal earlier.** Can you eat your last meal in the early evening to allow plenty of time for digestion before bedtime? Our gut bacteria benefits from a 12-hour rest from digesting food.[96] It's hard work breaking down food, and giving them at least 12 hours off at night encourages more favourable changes to their populations in the gut.
- ❀ **Snack if you need to.** If you ignore the feeling and become ravenous, you're more likely to overeat or grab a less healthy choice.
- ❀ **Do an evening check-in.** Many of us snack in the evening to curb feelings of boredom, or sometimes of loneliness and stress. Can you decide if it's hunger or something else? Could you grab a favourite book, call

a friend for a chat or sip a (decaffeinated) hot drink or water instead? Are you thirsty?

✽ **Lower your alcohol intake.** The health risks of excess alcohol drinking are well established (it increases the risk of high blood pressure, heart disease, stroke, liver disease, cancers and digestive issues like heartburn).[97] And for our gut health, the best amount of alcohol is . . . zero. It can also increase our risk of anxiety and sleep issues.[98,99] Many people are realising that not drinking is having a dramatic, positive impact on their physical, mental and emotional health. Whether you're cutting back or stopping, you can seek support and inspiration from online forums and meet-ups if that helps.

Combat the bloat

This is THE most common issue I see when people increase the amount of healthy plant foods in their diet. These foods are so important for long-term health, but when you run into trouble with bloating, wind and tummy pains, the last thing you'll want to do is eat more beans!

Meat, fish and refined carbohydrates like white flour are mostly digested by your enzymes higher up in the gut. Plant foods are mostly digested by your gut bacteria. To be able to enjoy your plant foods without discomfort you will need: 1) microbes in your gut that have the enzymes you need to digest plants and 2) a relaxed gut.

When you suddenly increase the fibre content of your foods, your digestive system is not ready. You haven't yet built up those populations of gut microbes needed to avoid the bloat. Don't worry, this doesn't do you any harm, but it can be uncomfortable. Equally, when you are anxious or stressed, or if you have recently had antibiotics or a tummy bug – your gut–brain–microbiota axis can be off kilter. This means your gut is less efficient at absorbing the gas your gut bugs produce when digesting fibre.

Tips for adopting a plant-based diet

- ❀ **If you currently don't eat a plant-based diet, start slowly so as not to shock your system.** If you're feeling uncomfortable, start with a tablespoon of beans or a quarter of the fruit that you think is causing your discomfort, and do this for a few weeks. As your body adjusts, you can increase your intake of that food.
- ❀ **Soaking uncooked beans overnight and then rinsing them thoroughly before cooking** helps reduce the gas your gut bugs make while digesting the beans. Cook them well. If your beans are already precooked in a can or carton, rinse them until the liquid runs clear without bubbling. This reduces the risk of gas in your gut from consuming the oligosaccharides, proteins and saponins that have leaked into the water from storing in the can or carton.
- ❀ **Try tofu, tempeh and hummus.** These are all legumes with fewer fermentable carbohydrates.
- ❀ **Prebiotic supplements can help feed those beneficial gut bugs**, and they're especially useful if you are someone who bloats. Examples include beta glucans (found in oats, barley, seaweed and certain types of mushrooms), psyllium husk and acacia powder. Remember: start low (one dose with a meal) and slow (one at a time) to build up the benefits.

❀ **If you're struggling, digestive enzymes can give you a helping hand** before a bean-rich meal. They can be bought online or from health food shops.

❀ **Belly breathing** – yes, it really works! Engaging the parasympathetic nervous system can improve digestion. If you're not sure how, put your hand on your stomach and breathe in for four seconds so your stomach stretches like a soft balloon, and your chest stays still. Hold it for two seconds, gently breathe out for four and don't breathe in again for two.

❀ **Ginger tea helps with nausea; peppermint and chamomile help to relax your smooth muscle** (what your gut is made from) and fennel gets things moving through if you are feeling constipated.

❀ **Try a gentle walk** after your meal to help your stomach empty.

If you find it helpful, keep a food diary to figure out which foods may be associated with gastrointestinal symptoms. It may also help you to know what your usual food habits are and how they could impact your energy levels, sleep and exercise routines.

When to seek help

If you have symptoms like persistent bloating, weight loss, bleeding from the bottom and blood in your poo, abdominal pain, acid reflux, black poo, pale poo, tiredness or any change in bowel habit, please see your doctor for further tests.

If you are diagnosed with irritable bowel syndrome (IBS), you may find a healthy, wholefoods, plant-based diet improves your symptoms dramatically. However, some people notice bloating and pain increases at first when they try to up their fibre intake. There are many things you can do to address IBS that do not involve food. For example, exercise like yoga (which combines movement, weight-bearing exercise and mindfulness) can be really helpful.[100] Talking therapies are also useful (as we know, there is a strong connection between our brains and our bodies, see pages 4 and 148). Often when my patients have tried everything, one of the things they did not know is that trauma, PTSD and anxiety are linked to digestive issues and lack of gut-microbe diversity.[101]

Lastly, when it comes to food, many people with IBS get relief from a short-term FODMAP diet. FODMAP is an acronym that stands for fermentable oligosaccharides, disaccharides, monosaccharides and polyols. It is a mouthful. It basically means simple sugars that are linked together and are fermentable by our gut bugs. These simple sugars pull water into the gut. The qualities of FODMAP-rich foods can lead to flatulence and loose stools. Wind is a combination of methane, hydrogen and carbon dioxide, and methane can slow gut motility and contribute to constipation. So, bloating from FODMAP sensitivity can then be a result of a combination of solids (hard poo), liquids (soft poo) and gases (wind) in the gut. Eliminating FODMAPs seems logical, and has in fact been shown in clinical trials to improve IBS symptoms.[102]

However, FODMAP-rich foods are also prebiotics, meaning they help healthy gut bugs to thrive. They have other health benefits too. For example, avocados can increase absorption of antioxidants in food, apples can improve weight maintenance, watermelons and garlic can improve blood pressure and beans can lower blood cholesterol. So how can we get the sweet spot of health benefits without the bloat?

If you gradually reintroduce certain high-FODMAP foods after restriction, digestive symptoms can be relieved and beneficial gut bugs can thrive at the same time. Think of this process like going to the gym to build strong muscles. If you are not primed, you would not lift the heaviest weights for fear of injury.

Instead, you'd start slowly and gradually increase the weights you lift. In the same way, if you have a FODMAP intolerance you need to restrict, observe and gradually work back in the foods that caused your symptoms. Get the support of a registered nutritionist or dietician to do this, and if you are not in a position for that, a great start would be to look at the 'GROWTH' strategy by Dr Will Bulsiewicz, as described in his book *The Fibre Fuelled Cookbook*.[103]

Food anxiety and eating disorders

I am fed up with diets. My patients are fed up with diets. On the flip side, who hasn't reached for a glass of wine, a pint, a bag of crisps or a chocolate bar to satisfy a craving or get an immediate feeling of calm or pleasure? I know I have. Unfortunately, when we are low, we are far more likely to reach for alcohol, salt, sugar and fat than a plate of broccoli.

This is partly because we are hardwired to crave calorie-dense foods. But mainly it's because manufactured foods are designed so we crave them – the perfect balance of sugar, fat, salt, emulsifiers, crunch and melt-in-the-mouth textures to please our taste buds and stimulate the release of metabolic, stress, and appetite hormones – insulin, cortisol, dopamine, leptin and ghrelin – all of which play a role in cravings.[104]

Have you ever felt guilty for eating a 'bad' food? Perhaps you've felt anxiety around food, as well as guilt? Have you calorie-counted every meal and upped your exercise to atone for less healthy food choices?

For many, these patterns can easily spiral, resulting in stress when thinking about food, and in feeling bad about themselves.

Developing bulimia nervosa or anorexia nervosa are outward signs of an eating disorder, but there is danger in behavioural eating patterns that fall outside of these diagnoses as well. I had a patient (we will call her Amelia) who was heavily into sports at school, and her mum brought her in to see me, as Amelia was withdrawing into herself and not eating with the rest of the family. Mum reported that she had become preoccupied with healthy eating, reading books on nutrition and refusing to eat anything that had any fat, including salad dressings, nuts and seeds. She was in Year 11 and was struggling to concentrate during her exams, and had fainted on her way to one of the end-of-school tests. I spoke to Amelia alone, and she was low in mood. She had stopped taking part in hockey. She wanted to be as thin as her friends and was following so-called 'pro-ana' and 'pro-mia' social media accounts (promoting anorexia and bulimia as lifestyle choices, rather than illnesses). Although she was presenting with a normal body weight, it was clear Amelia was developing disordered eating patterns and struggling with her mood as a result. I referred her to local mental health support services as well as the resources of Beat, the UK's eating disorder charity. With family support, she was able to regain the energy she needed to get through her exams, restart her hockey practice in college and access the help she needed.

Disordered eating is often about your inner experience – you can be any age, sex, weight or shape, with a successful career or family life, and still experience disordered eating because of how food and eating makes you feel. For many of us, it can be hard to be surrounded by impossible ideals of physical perfection and skinniness, or the perfect muscular physique. This is made all the more difficult when we compare ourselves to what we see on the TV, or scrolling through social media. Airbrushed perfection. But could plant-based eating – or specifically veganism – be a part of the problem too?

Disordered eating is something that can become pervasive for anyone, and could also contribute to problems with self-esteem and our relationship with food. So it is an important part of the puzzle when we talk about what being healthy and plant-based means.

The image of veganism in the media is often one of skinny, tanned, cucumber-water-drinking, yoga-posing young white women. The people I see in clinic are often very different from this. My patients are struggling with chronic diseases and looking for tools they can use to improve them. I see men in their seventies with high blood pressure; women in their fifties trying to cope with menopausal symptoms; men in their forties struggling with excess weight; women in their twenties with endometriosis – people who want practical solutions to their health issues.

One of the benefits of a plant-based diet is that when you are eating predominantly fruits, vegetables, wholegrains and pulses, nuts and seeds, you have a nutrient-, water- and fibre-rich eating pattern. It is easier to fill up on these foods without taking in as many calories (or as much energy) and therefore it is easier to lose excess weight (if that is the goal). Eating this way is linked to reduced risk of being overweight, having type 2 diabetes and reducing overall cancer risk too.[105-107]

But what if 'veganism' was a way of avoiding family dinners, meals out with friends or even became a source of constant pre-occupation? What if – even subconsciously – veganism is a way to make food restriction socially acceptable and to stop people from asking questions about why you are not eating? There is a term for excessive focus on only eating healthy foods – orthorexia – and sometimes veganism and orthorexia can overlap.

Orthorexia can occur with many different diets – and although it is not officially a mental illness in the DSM (*Diagnostic and Statistical Manual of Mental Disorders*, published by the American

Psychiatric Association and used worldwide), it can be a psychologically harmful pattern of thinking, and is worth understanding. Think about how it might feel to become so focused on whether you are eating healthily enough to achieve your ideas of outward perfection: enough salads to get that flat stomach, enough kale smoothies to lose those extra layers of cellulite. Enough healthy choices to look worthy of love, success, happiness. When this focus mutates into an obsession, it becomes an illness.

Many experts believe that vegan and vegetarian diets can increase the risk of eating disorders. Some treatment centres consider the reintroduction of meat a necessary part of recovery. These beliefs are based on data that reported higher rates of disordered eating among vegetarians compared to nonvegetarians.[108-113] Currently, about half of young women with anorexia eat some form of vegetarian diet, whereas only 6 to 34 per cent of their non-anorexic peers eat a vegetarian diet.[114] Although you might logically conclude that vegetarian diets *cause* eating disorders, evidence indicates that vegetarian diets are typically started *after* onset and often mask eating disorders. In other words, vegetarian diets are embarked upon as part of a pattern to facilitate food restriction and cause loved ones to ask fewer questions about the removal of high-fat animal products and fast foods made with these products.[115,116] One research team called this 'pseudovegetarianism'.[116] This does not mean that vegetarians can't develop eating disorders. It also does not mean that people with eating disorders won't decide to become vegetarian for other reasons while they're ill or recovering. Both possibilities exist.

It really helps to ask yourself: 'Why am I eating this way?'

A 2012 study of 160 women examined their motivation for becoming vegetarian. Almost half the participants with a history of eating disorders mentioned weight concerns as a main motivation for becoming vegetarian. In the control group, *none* of the vegetarian participants became vegetarian because of concerns about body weight.[113] In 2012, two research papers provided valuable insights into the link between vegetarianism and eating disorders. The first paper reported that semi-vegetarians (who didn't eat red meat) and flexitarians (who had occasional red-meat consumption) were significantly *more* restrained in their eating habits than omnivores or vegetarians.[117] In addition, the fewer animal products the vegetarians ate (in other words, the more vegan they became), the *less* likely they were to exhibit signs of disordered eating.

The authors noted that while the semi-vegetarians and flexitarians were motivated by weight concerns, vegetarians and pescatarians were motivated by ethical concerns. The second paper (which included two separate studies) carefully separated vegetarians and vegans.[118] The investigators also found that vegans had the healthiest scores of all dietary groups and speculated that vegan diets may actually be *protective* against developing eating disorders.[118] The conclusions makes some sense, given that many vegans have external motivation (their concern for animals and the environment) as opposed to the internally focused motivation of losing weight.

What about overeating?

There are many reasons why we might eat more than we need, just as there are many reasons why we might restrict our food. In fact, when we restrict eating behaviours for the sake of weight loss, there are complex physiological responses at play to help our body to regain lost weight.[119] Diets just don't seem to work.[120] Eighty per cent of dieters regain lost weight within five years.[121] This is nothing to do with willpower. Weight loss is accompanied by persistent hormone adaptations that increase appetite and decrease satiety (fullness), which causes the body to resist continued efforts at weight loss.[122] Furthermore, a relatively persistent effort is required to avoid overeating to match the increased appetite that grows in proportion to the weight lost.[123,124] In other words, it is hard and it is not your fault.

We become naturally drawn to salty, sugary or high-energy foods for all sorts of reasons. Gaining comfort from food is an absolutely normal human tendency. When food is more abundant and energy-dense than at any other time in human existence, it makes sense that many of us struggle with being overweight. Processed foods simply did not exist before industrial-scale food systems. High-energy-dense and low-nutrient-dense cakes, crisps, pastries, sweets, fizzy pop and ice cream are brand new, when we think in terms of the last few hundred thousand years of human development. The food industry spends many millions on scientific research to hijack our taste buds and brains to make foods as palatable as possible, to keep us wanting more. The odds are definitely stacked against us. To feel bad about yourself for eating this food is unhelpful, and completely misplaced.

You might find it surprising to hear me say this, but becoming overweight is actually, for the most part, outside of our conscious control. Take budget, for starters. Food insecurity – not knowing if you can afford your next meal – can cause people to eat more than they normally would when they get the chance, and less than they normally would if they cannot afford to.[125] In places where it is harder to buy healthy, nutritious food, people are also exposed to more advertising for fast food. They are also surrounded by more fast-food outlets.[126] Buying unhealthy food then becomes more of a logical decision. Having the time, flexibility, finances and social support to listen to your body and make nutritious food is a real privilege.

In December 2022, The Trussell Trust food-bank network in the

UK distributed an emergency food parcel to someone every eight seconds and, for the first time, had to give out more than was being donated.[127] So many people – including those with full-time jobs – are struggling to make ends meet. Intense financial stress can itself increase waist size, as your cortisol levels rise. Stress and lack of sleep caused by a chronic health condition can also be linked to weight gain. Our emotions, a history of abuse as a child, life traumas – all of these and more can affect our chances of being obese as adults. In fact, a meta-analysis of studies on this issue concluded there was a 46 per cent increase in the odds of someone experiencing adult obesity if they had been exposed to many adverse events in childhood.[128] So, you will see that our body size is heavily influenced by many factors that are outside of our control – even before we have picked up an item of food from the shop and taken it home.

What is the answer to over- and undereating?

Self-compassion (as explored in the chapter Love) is the root of understanding and accepting who we are, and what we really want. So often, we are triggered by a feeling, or something external, which makes us want to change how we feel as quickly as possible. Then, bingeing, purging or severe restriction of food can make you feel worse.[129] In her book *The Last Diet*, behavioural change scientist Shahroo Izadi talks about how remembering that an urge to eat something is more of a 'yoo-hoo' from your brain than a 'must-do'. Notice it. Pause for a moment and ask yourself if your most trusted friend or someone that you respect and look up to would advise you to eat whatever snack you are craving in that moment. It is a surprisingly useful mental exercise in understanding if your desire for a food is matched by your physical hunger, or if it is coming from a place of boredom or discomfort.

As for dietary patterns, there is no one 'quick fix' diet for ideal weight balance. The 'diet' that works is the lifestyle you can keep.[130] There are so many reasons to eat a more plant-based diet. People turn to it for its health benefits, its lower carbon footprint, its kindness towards animals or simply for its encouragement to eat more veggies. If plant-based living has been triggering for you, or your motivation is based around only weight loss or looking good, it might not be the healthiest choice psychologically. Otherwise, don't let fear of disordered eating be a reason to avoid a plant-based lifestyle, because for many it offers a chance to practise compassion for themselves as well as for the planet.

I'd like to share the story of Adam Sud, who struggled with food addiction, and who found a way to heal through self-compassion. A few years ago, Adam's life consisted mostly of sitting on his sofa, surrounded by fast-food wrappers and looking for his next fix. He was addicted to prescription painkillers and was suffering from severe depression. He weighed 22st 12lb (145kg) at the time. Reflecting on this, he said:

> I was miserable all the time. I hated my life, myself, and blamed everyone else for my situation. I was never comfortable in any social situation and I was constantly self-conscious about my weight. I had spent everything I had on drugs, food and impulse online buys. I thought I had reached rock bottom when I overdosed. But then I woke up, surrounded by fast-food wrappers and mess. I called my parents for help and went to rehab two weeks later. It was there that I was diagnosed with type 2 diabetes, high cholesterol and high blood pressure.

Adam decided to include plant-based nutrition in his recovery programme of medication and therapy. What he didn't realise at the time was that his diet changes would become the backbone of his entire recovery. Within three months Adam had reversed his diabetes, normalised his cholesterol and stabilised his blood pressure. Within a year he was able to come off his medications, including his mood stabilisers and antidepressants. Since then, Adam also discovered the joys of sober living and fitness. He lost 14 stone (89kg) and decided to dedicate his life to helping others through addiction recovery. He became a fitness coach and nutritionist, and now runs his own programmes teaching nutrition as part of recovery at outpatient therapy centres. Adam not only learned to love and respect the body he has, but he also changed his identity. He became someone focused on self-compassion and helping other people with similar struggles.

Incredibly, Adam also became an author in the recent 'INFINITE' study, the first controlled trial to investigate the impact of nutrition education on early addiction-recovery outcomes. In the trial, both groups received weekly nutrition education sessions to complement their recovery. One group was given plant-based foods, while the other group was given the standard American diet as a control. At ten weeks the plant-based group experienced significant increases in resilience and self-esteem compared to the control group.[131] These are two powerful factors in predicting long-term recovery from addiction. Adam and his team of researchers hope more efforts to include nutrition into the support of people with addictions can be made. He said:

> I want to help people take charge of their lives with simple, affordable food choices. For your mental health, seek out a support group, a therapist or a psychiatrist, someone who can help you figure out the next steps. And remember: you are not broken because you feel. You feel because you are whole. I know what it's like to struggle with health issues,

and I know how hard it can feel. Let me be the one to tell you it's worth it. You are worth it.

What does 'food freedom' look like?

Consume a healthy and broad range of foods – in a plant-based diet, this should include nuts, seeds, nut butters, avocados, tofu, legumes, starchy vegetables and wholegrains. For those focused on health, don't be afraid of the occasional vegan junk-food option. Enjoy it if you want it – no guilt, please.

Avoid giving foods moral value – 'good' or 'bad'. Eating cake on a birthday is not 'bad'. Perhaps instead think about nutrients in food; and yes, it is true some foods have more energy and fewer nutrients than others.

Portion sizes: try not to compare your portion to someone else's, or limit your portion size based on what a plate 'should' look like. Sometimes you are not very hungry and only need a piece of toast, other times a large meal and seconds is what you need. Remember to take your time and connect with the food you're enjoying; appreciate it. This will help you to know how much you need. If you are not used to following hunger cues, I urge you to read Shahroo Izadi's *The Last Diet* for more specific tips on how to regulate your eating patterns in a healthy and sustainable way.

Remember, we cannot all be responsible for all of our food choices all of the time. Do not judge others for what they eat – or yourself.

If you have a history of disordered eating, you may want to avoid intermittent fasting. Although this is a useful tool for some, for others it can be hard to trust hunger cues again when you externally regulate when you should eat. There are not many studies on intermittent fasting for premenopausal women. If you're not getting regular periods, intermittent fasting can be a way to disconnect from your body and try to control it – which makes food struggles harder. Instead, perhaps aim to avoid snacking after dinner if you want to extend your window of eating, as this will support your circadian rhythm and your ability to digest your food (as discussed in the Sleep chapter).

Women – it is okay and indeed normal to wobble! A flat stomach, extremely lean thighs and low body fat percentage could mean you lose your periods. Having a period is a sign of health and fertility in premenopausal women. If what society has told you is the right 'look' means you don't have periods, it is not healthy for you. You'll have to sit somewhere in the range of 21 to 33 per cent body fat to have a period, depending on your genes and build.

If you are tempted to binge eat, try delaying the impulse to act – even by five minutes. This can apply to eating foods, but also to any situation which causes us to immediately respond negatively. Delay tactics give you a chance to rethink or evaluate what your ideal response would be in a situation. Don't think of it as 'impulse control' but rather as 'impulse recognition' and even 'impulse compassion'.

Move your body because it feels good, not as a punishment or to 'make up for' what you ate or what you are about to eat. If you have been successful in losing excess weight, exercise is also a great way of ensuring that your ideal weight is maintained by your healthier lifestyle. Physical activity is great for reducing risk of cancers, muscle loss, cognitive decline and balance problems as you get older. There are so many more reasons to exercise than losing weight!

Remember that you are enough. You are not broken. You are a miraculous human, and worthy of your own love. Health does not equate to worth and neither does slimness; think about what makes you feel important, valued and loved.

Be honest with someone you trust – you can't feel seen unless you allow yourself to be seen. If you have hidden disordered eating and are ready to seek help, contact a friend, loved one, your doctor or a clinic for help.

Dr Tara Kemp is a mental health researcher (lead author on the 'INFINITE' study), and her doctorate research was on the topic of eating disorder recovery. Her evidence-based approach to eating disorder recovery focuses on self-compassion. She has kindly shared her story here and shares how she turned food from a form of self-harm to one of self-love.

I first started struggling with food when I was about 14 years old. Like many people, it wasn't body image that led me down that road. Sure, I grew up in a patriarchal world where diet culture is the norm, so I received the same messages as every other female that a thinner body was a better body. Additionally, up until that point, I'd been a gymnast, so I was regularly complimented on my muscle tone as well. It's not surprising that the eating disorder developed when I stopped being a gymnast – and amidst puberty, found my body changing in ways that I'd learned were undesirable.

But just as body image is a surface-level view of a person, it is a surface-level view of disordered eating as well. The true issue at hand was that I was feeling lost and alone. I was experiencing an identity crisis. I felt shame about my anxiety, and the world felt out of my control. When we don't have healthy tools and skills to support us in coping with uncomfortable emotions and experiences, we turn to something else that can provide us with a sense of control or distraction. Like many, I turned to food.

When I was struggling with my own disordered eating as a teenager, most of the guidance I received was not helpful for my recovery. This is because many of the physicians and dieticians that I saw were trained within the standard medical model, which works to reduce or eliminate the symptoms of a condition. So while I increased my food intake, restored my weight to a healthy BMI range, and regained my period (albeit through a birth control prescription), the root causes of the condition were never fully addressed.

When I decided to adopt a plant-based lifestyle over a decade ago, my family saw this as a resurgence of the eating disorder. Their perspective was aligned with the majority of experts within the eating disorder field at that time. Veganism was seen as a form of disordered eating – a socially acceptable method of restriction and control. But the situation wasn't as simple as it appeared; I actually found myself feeling less stressed about eating the 'right' thing, and more connected to the driving values behind my food choices. Although it looked like restriction, I had in fact found a sense of freedom in these mindful eating guidelines. Eating was embedded with meaning and purpose.

I am not alone in this experience. Although research is limited, there are multiple studies showing that people following a vegan diet actually have a healthier relationship with food in comparison to other forms of vegetarianism, and even in comparison to omnivores.[117,118] In addition to reading the science, I can relate to my personal experience and the experience of my clients as well. I now get huge satisfaction from doing this work as a career. I help people to build a toolbox of the recovery model components: a meaningful life, a connection to self, supportive relationships and a positive self-identity. And when it comes to veganism, if the motive is based in values that help someone to act more in alignment with who they are, and if the lifestyle brings someone a sense of meaning and purpose, it may in fact be the healthiest way forward for their ultimate recovery.

Being able to get on with, and even admire, the person you are is the greatest gift you can give to yourself, and sets the tone for all the other interactions and relationships you have. Taking 30 minutes to write down promises you want to keep to yourself when you are in a hard place mentally is a really valuable exercise. I call them 'vows' to give them more gravity, and to recognise that trusting myself is a bit like a sacred promise.

Personal promises

I was so moved hearing about Tara's journey and how she now gets so much satisfaction from helping others enjoy their relationship with food again. Are there any promises that you would like to keep when thinking about your own health, or your own happiness? Are there any patterns of thinking that have held you back that you'd like to let go of? If so, make some new promises to yourself that feel right for you. Keep them in your journal or the notes on your phone, for when you need a reminder of what's important to you.

How to start eating more plants

What do you need to buy to get started? What do you already own that will serve you well? As you flick through some of the recipes, you may be pleasantly surprised at how much you already own, such as oats, fruit, rice, pasta, beans and herbs. Go and have a look in your cupboards, and see what you already have before you order online or head down to the shops.

Quick and easy recipes

If you have some fast, go-to meals to turn to that you can also freeze and defrost for the week ahead, it makes the switch to a wholefoods, plant-based diet feel a bit easier. All the recipes here take less than 30 minutes to make.

There are lots of brilliant cookbooks to turn to for further inspiration and I've listed my favourites in the resources section.

In my first book, I also included 60 recipes for breakfast, lunch, dinner and snacks that made family-favourite comfort foods, like mac 'n' cheese and spaghetti bolognese, wholefoods and plant-based to show how you can still eat what you love and reduce your saturated fat, meat, fish and dairy intake. This time I wanted to focus on speed and affordability, which can feel like barriers to making any diet change.

In this recipes section, I have some wonderful ideas for you - not just from my kitchen, but from the kitchens of some truly amazing pioneers in the world of wellness. I'm fortunate to be part of a community of like-minded people whom I also call good friends. They have each shared a bit about their story, and which aspects of the GLOVES framework have been important to them. They have kindly donated their own favourites to get your mouth watering!

I include a QR code opposite so you can see some of these delicious recipes brought to life. Hopefully it will inspire you even further to give these amazing dishes a try!

There are 18 recipes here: quick breakfasts, easy snacks, simple soups and salads (I love these for my work lunchbox/flask) and fast and filling mains. My kids love all these recipes and I enjoy being able to throw these together after a busy day in clinic.

A note on ingredients: there are some expensive ingredients here among the fresh, tinned and store cupboard staples. I include them for their nutritional importance and flavour, but I am mindful that they might feel like more of an investment, so I have made sure to reuse them in all the recipes to make the most of each.

Quick breakfasts

Banana Crepes with Raspberry Compote

I personally adore crepes – my childhood memories are of thin, crispy pancakes with lemon and sugar. It was the ultimate treat! This recipe scratches that itch, but the banana adds a caramel twist that I really like.

Makes 6 crepes
You'll need: a whisk, a non-stick pan and a ladle

For the crepes
1 tsp vegan butter or oil,
  for frying
1 cup plain flour
1 tbsp ground flaxseed
1 cup any plant milk
1 very ripe banana

For the compote
1 cup frozen raspberries
1 tsp sugar
1 tsp cornflour

For the topping
Spoonful of coconut cream
  or yoghurt
Maple syrup (optional)

1. Blend the flour, flaxseed, plant milk and banana to make a batter.

2. In a non-stick pan, melt 1 teaspoon of vegan butter or oil over medium heat.

3. Put a ladleful of the batter in the pan and move the pan around, distributing the batter evenly to make a thin crepe.

4. After the crepe has cooked for a couple of minutes, flip it over and cook on the other side for 1 to 2 minutes, until lightly golden.

5. Pile up the crepes on a warm plate as you cook them, or place a kitchen cloth over them to retain the heat.

6. Meanwhile, in a small saucepan, make your compote: add the frozen raspberries, sugar and cornflour to a pan, with a dash of water, and stir until the raspberries disintegrate and the

Continues opposite

liquid turns thick (as the cornflour cooks).

7. Remove from heat. Serve crepes with the compote over the top, a dollop of coconut cream or yoghurt, and maple syrup if you like. Perfect!

Breakfast Berry Smoothie

. . . .

I make this for a quick snack. If you want to have it for breakfast,
I'd recommend adding some protein to keep you full – you can use
soy or pea milk instead of water or another plant milk (as they have
a higher protein content than other plant milks); a scoop of vegan
protein powder; a tablespoon of flaxseed, chia seeds or hemp
seeds; or a dollop of almond butter, peanut butter or tahini would
all be delicious – use what you have to hand.

Protein powders often taste of things like chocolate, vanilla or
salted caramel – so if you decide to add this, your smoothie easily
acts as a dessert too. My kids love it served in a bowl with fresh fruit,
a nut butter, granola and desiccated coconut or nuts/seeds on top.

With smoothies, I'd advise you to get green leafy veggies in to
reduce sugar and increase variety and nutrients. Top up with
unsweetened plant milk or water instead of juice if you want a
thinner consistency. If you need to fuel an intense exercise schedule, you can add things like dried fruit, nut and seed butters, and
oats to increase the energy density. Experiment and have fun!

Makes 2 portions
You'll need: a freezer and a blender

*2–3 cups unsweetened
soy milk*
1 sprig frozen kale
1 frozen banana, halved
*1 handful mixed frozen
berries*
*⅓ a cucumber, thickly
chopped*
*½ a carrot, thickly
chopped*
3 large pitted dates

1. If you don't have any frozen fruit or
veg, pop the ingredients you need in
the freezer the night before. This helps
to make the smoothie colder and
brings out the sweetness in the banana.

2. Add all the ingredients to a blender
and blend until thick and smooth.
Serve!

Overnight Oats

. . . .

This doesn't require cooking – you just leave oats and a plant milk mixed together overnight to do their thing, and you have a delicious and healthy breakfast the next morning. If you want it sooner, it will take around half an hour to absorb the milk. Also known as Bircher muesli, this takes a couple of minutes to prepare and can last 2 to 3 days in the fridge. The secret is your added ingredients! I love adding chia seeds to mine as a base, and I also put a tea bag in (my favourite is chai) to give a delicious flavour the next morning.

Makes 2 portions

You'll need: a large bowl (and a portable glass jar, if eating on the go)

1 cup gluten-free or regular rolled oats
1 cup plant milk
4 tbsp chia seeds
2 tbsp maple syrup

Optional extras
2 teaspoons of chopped nuts of your choice
2 teaspoons of desiccated coconut
¼ tsp vanilla extract
¼ tsp cinnamon
2 tbsp nut butter
20g raisins
20g pumpkin seeds
20g dried mango
20g flaked almonds
A pinch of cardamom

1. Mix your oats, chia seeds, maple syrup and plant milk together in a large bowl and be sure to submerge all the oats and seeds fully.

2. Add any of the extras, if desired.

3. Pop in the fridge overnight or for at least 30 minutes. Decant a portion into a glass jar to take with you, if you like.

Katie White's Story and Recipe

Katie White is the author of *The Seasonal Vegan* cookbook and is a Le Cordon Bleu–trained plant-based chef, photographer and musician. For Katie, plant-based cooking stemmed from her love of animals and her connection to nature. Being outdoors and discovering the medicinal and culinary value of the plants that surround her are the things that give her the most meaning when she looks at her own GLOVES framework. Katie says:

Growing up in rural Western Australia, I was lucky enough to have a childhood surrounded by animals of all kinds, from horses to hens, rescued lambs, kangaroos and everything in between. As a child I even adopted an injured lizard who became a loving companion! I began to feel a deep love and care for the animals and the rhythms of the natural world around me.

In my early twenties I found veganism as a way of life that caused the least harm to animals, and I realised that eating a plant-based diet was a way to align my everyday actions with what my heart told me. When I learned about the health benefits and reduced impact on the planet, it was a lovely bonus and fuelled my desire to make plants delicious so others could love this lifestyle as much as I do.

I decided to learn from the best and trained with Le Cordon Bleu. It is wonderful to know that my future life's work will be for the animals, in a way that humans can benefit from too.

Katie's Blueberry, Lemon and Hemp Seed Muffins

· ·

These muffins can be made for a treat breakfast or mid-morning snack, enjoyed with a mid-afternoon cuppa or perhaps made for a picnic with family.

They are perfectly fluffy and not too sweet; these muffins are loved by everyone and a great way to sneak a serving of omega-3-rich hemp seeds into your diet. The lemon zest gives the ultimate citrus notes to balance sweet blueberries.

Makes 9 large or 12 medium muffins
You'll need: a muffin pan, a whisk, two large bowls

2 cups plain flour
1 ½ tsp baking powder
¾ cup caster sugar
2 tbsp hemp seeds
   (preferably unhulled)
¾ cup plant milk
⅓ cup neutral oil
   (e.g. grapeseed)
6 drops food-grade
   lemon essential oil,
   or the zest of a
   lemon
1 tbsp vanilla extract
1 ½ cups blueberries

1. Whisk together the flour, baking powder, sugar and hemp seeds in a large bowl, then stir through the blueberries.

2. In another bowl, whisk together the milk, oil, essential oil or lemon zest and vanilla essence.

3. Fold the wet and dry mixes together gently (do not overmix or the muffin will be less fluffy). Then scoop 3–4 tablespoons of the mix into each muffin case (a lever ice cream scoop is ideal for this) and bake in the oven at 180°C/350°F/gas mark 4 for 25 minutes or until lightly browned on top.

Easy snacks

Apricot, Tahini and Coconut Balls

· ·

I love these with a cup of tea – they are packed full of vitamins and calcium, and are a good snack for kids' lunchboxes on days out, and for travel if you need something easy.

Makes 20 balls
You'll need: a food processor or blender

1 cup dried apricots
1 cup desiccated coconut (and extra for rolling – optional)
½ cup large, soft medjool dates
1 carrot, finely grated (not peeled)
1 tbsp chia seeds
4 tbsp tahini
½ cup raw cashew nuts, pistachios or almonds
1 tbsp water
1 tsp vanilla extract
A pinch of sea salt
A pinch of cinnamon, cardamom and ginger (optional)
A dash of maple syrup (optional)

1. Add the dates and apricots to the food processor and pulse for a minute until finely chopped.
2. Add the desiccated coconut, carrot, nuts, water, chia seeds, vanilla extract, maple syrup, salt and spices. Blitz them until they are a coarse mixture.
3. Add 4 tablespoons of tahini and mix. If the texture feels too dry and crumbly, add tahini. If it's too wet, add coconut.
4. Scoop a tablespoon of the mixture and roll it into a ball in your palm – this is the fun part!
5. Roll each of the balls in the remaining desiccated coconut.
6. Chill in the fridge for at least an hour before serving, and they will last for up to a week (or longer if you freeze them).

Chocolate-date Bites

· ·

These are ridiculously simple and delicious – a treat if you fancy something sweet with your cuppa or as a mid-afternoon snack. You could scale this up and make a batch in advance for the week, with as many dates as you have – a pack usually has around 16 dates, so have a jar of almond butter handy.

Makes 1 serving
You'll need: a saucepan and a heatproof bowl

1 soft medjool date
1 tsp almond butter
20g dark chocolate
(2–3 squares),
melted
Flaky sea salt

1. Gently cut your date lengthways and remove the stone.
2. Spoon a teaspoon of almond butter inside. Leave to one side on some parchment.
3. Melt the chocolate in a bowl set over a pan of boiling water, and stir it as it melts.
4. Once melted, carefully remove the chocolate from the heat and either pour over the date or dip it in the chocolate.
5. Sprinkle with the sea salt.

Simple swaps

You can swap the sea salt for dried cranberry, dried raspberry or sesame seeds for a more blood pressure-friendly snack.

Simple soups and salads

Green Goodness Soup

· ·

This is one of my favourite soups. It is one of my mum's recipes and so has the added home-comfort factor for me! It's tasty and filling and has a unique flavour. I freeze it in batches and take it out when I need it; the flavour isn't spoilt after freezing. If you've got a soup maker, you can add all the ingredients except for the second tin of butter beans. Add the second tin after the soup is cooked, for added texture.

Makes 5 portions (or about 8 starter portions)
You'll need: a large saucepan and a stick blender

1 medium onion, chopped
4 cloves garlic, chopped
150g frozen spinach, defrosted
250g broccoli florets
3 level tsp cumin powder
½ tsp cumin seeds
30g fresh parsley, chopped
2 x 400g tin of butter beans, drained and thoroughly rinsed
1 tbsp lemon juice
400ml tin of coconut milk
2 vegetable stock cubes
300ml water
Salt and pepper, to taste

1. In a saucepan on medium heat, put the onion, garlic, spinach, broccoli, cumin powder, cumin seeds, parsley, 1 can of butter beans, lemon juice, coconut milk, stock cubes, water, and salt and pepper to taste.

2. Bring to the boil and simmer for 30 minutes.

3. Using the stick blender, blend the soup in the saucepan, leaving some bits unblended if you wish to give it more texture.

4. Add the second tin of washed and drained butter beans, for additional texture.

5. Serve straight away. However, this soup builds even better flavour when it's been left for a day in the fridge and then heated up.

Hearty, Warming Tomato Soup

. . . .

A thick, hearty and gorgeous soup. You'll notice that I've not included any oil to fry the onions in at the beginning – there is no difference in taste, and if you have weight-loss goals, it makes sense to avoid the added oil. If you've got a soup maker, you can add all the ingredients and press start – but keep back the second tin of kidney beans to add afterwards for texture.

Makes 5 portions (or about 8 starter portions)
You'll need: a large saucepan and a stick blender

1 medium onion, chopped

3 cloves garlic, crushed

2 x 400g tin of chopped tomatoes

1 tsp cumin powder

4 tsp dried basil

1 tsp turmeric

400ml tin of coconut milk

200ml water

2 vegetable stock cubes

2 x 400g tin of kidney beans, drained and thoroughly rinsed

Salt and pepper, to taste

Optional basil leaves, to serve

1. Put the onion, garlic, tomatoes, cumin powder, dried basil, turmeric, coconut milk, water, vegetable stock cubes, one tin of kidney beans and salt and pepper into the saucepan.

2. Bring to the boil while stirring, then gently simmer for 30 minutes.

3. Blitz with the stick blender to desired consistency.

4. Add the second tin of kidney beans after blending, to add texture.

5. Serve with some fresh basil leaves on the top and a bread of choice if you wish, but I like it just as it is.

Ella Mills's Story and Recipe

Ella Mills is the creator of the bestselling *Deliciously Ella* cookbooks and brand, has six bestselling cookbooks, a plant-based food and wellness app, a huge range of food products in over 10,000 stores across the UK, a restaurant and a social media following of over 3 million people. But her journey to good health did not start out with these goals in mind. Thirteen years ago, she just wanted to get well. Ella began to have health issues at university; she had chronic fatigue, felt faint and extremely dizzy, suffered from heart palpitations and consistent pain and was bloated all the time, no matter what she did or didn't eat. She was eventually diagnosed with POTS (postural tachycardia syndrome) as well as Ehlers-Danlos syndrome (a connective tissue disorder) and mast cell activation syndrome, following many months in and out of hospital, desperate for answers. Ella says:

> The condition (POTS) affected the workings of my autonomic nervous system – I couldn't control my heart rate and blood pressure properly, while also struggling with digestive issues, chronic fatigue, a series of infections and a whole host of other symptoms. I was prescribed a cocktail of medication but unfortunately, they had limited success in managing the condition and after about a year, I hit rock bottom, both physically and mentally.
>
> It became clear that medication alone wasn't going to restore my health and I needed to do something else to help myself. At this point, I began researching whether a change in diet and lifestyle may be able to help. Encouraged by stories I read, I decided to turn to a wholefoods, plant-based diet. I had three major obstacles at this

point, though: 1) I couldn't cook and didn't really like vegetables; 2) I had no idea how to make plant-based recipes;
and 3) I had lost all of my sense of drive and self-esteem.

I decided the way to address all three issues was to start
a diary, pushing myself to try new things in the kitchen
each day, rediscover a sense of creativity and try to take
back a semblance of control when it came to my health.
So, I taught myself to cook and shared my findings on my
website deliciouslyella.com (deliciously because that was
always the goal – make healthy food delicious).

For me, healing was neither fast nor linear. A few
months into my new diet, I started to notice small glimpses
of hope, though – my brain fog had lessened, my joints
hurt a little less, my energy was ever so slightly better. That
gave me the inspiration I needed to keep going and, within
a few years, I was off all my daily medication and felt as
though I was thriving again.

The more I've learnt, the more I believe it's essential to
combine a healthy diet with a healthy lifestyle, beyond
what's on our plates. I really lean on other habits to keep
me on track physically and mentally – running a company
and having two young daughters certainly takes a lot out
of you, and it is easy to feel overwhelmed or anxious.
Meditation, yoga and time offline with my family are as
important to me as the food I cook now.

Many of Gemma's practical tips for getting well and
staying well have been truly foundational for me in my
journey towards health. I remember how challenging it
can feel to get started, and I want these changes to feel easy
for you. New habits are hard – but if we can make them
delicious, then I know from experience we are far more
likely to keep coming back to them.

Ella's Sweet Potato and Chickpea Salad

· ·

This has been my favourite salad for almost ten years. The sweet potatoes are tossed with cumin and paprika, then baked until tender, before being tossed with kale that's dressed with a creamy cashew dressing and finished with a sprinkling of fresh parsley, chilli flakes and black pepper. It's simple, creamy and delicious. Massaging kale may sound a little strange, but it makes a world of difference, softening the leaves to soak up maximum dressing.

Makes 4 portions

You'll need: a baking tray, a blender, a large mixing bowl and a vegetable peeler

For the salad

2 large sweet potatoes (500g), peeled and cut into bite-sized pieces

400g tin of chickpeas, drained and thoroughly rinsed

A drizzle of olive oil

1 tsp ground cumin

1 tsp paprika

200g kale, roughly chopped

1 handful fresh parsley, chopped

A pinch of sea salt

A pinch of black pepper

A pinch of dried red chilli flakes (optional, for a spicy kick!)

1. Preheat oven to 190°C/170°C fan/375°F/gas mark 5.

2. Place the sweet potato chunks and drained chickpeas onto a baking tray and drizzle with olive oil, cumin, paprika and a pinch of salt. Mix well and roast for 30 to 35 minutes, until the sweet potatoes begin to soften.

3. While they cook, make the dressing. Place all of the dressing ingredients into a powerful blender and blitz until smooth.

4. Place the kale into a large mixing bowl and add a drizzle of olive oil and a sprinkling of salt. Massage the kale with your hands for a few minutes, really rubbing the leaves until the kale is nice and soft. When

Continues opposite

For the dressing

150g cashews
2 cloves garlic, roasted
6 tbsp almond milk
1 tbsp nutritional yeast
  (optional)
2 tbsp Dijon mustard
Juice of 1 lemon
A pinch of sea salt

ready, pour over the dressing and gently rub it into the kale, again using your hands.

5. Once the sweet potatoes and chickpeas are cooked, remove from the oven. Allow to cool for a few minutes and then toss them through the kale.

6. Transfer to a serving bowl and finish with fresh parsley, a pinch of black pepper and a pinch of chilli flakes.

Fast mains

Teriyaki Noodles

. . . .

This simple dish takes just 15 minutes – it's flavoursome, quick and, best of all, easy to make. You can use wholewheat, buckwheat or brown rice noodles (the last two options are great if you need gluten-free noodles too). You can combine different colour peppers to increase your plant points!

Time-saving tip – either freeze your own crushed-up or grated ginger or garlic to use for later, or buy ready-frozen cubes from the shops to make the meal even quicker.

Makes 4 portions
You'll need: a saucepan, a wok and a strainer

For the noodles
200g noodles
A thumb of ginger, peeled and chopped
3 cloves garlic, peeled and chopped
200g oyster mushrooms (or your favourite mushroom)
1–2 spring onions
1 bunch pak choi
1 bell pepper, any colour
1 cup cashew nuts
½ a chilli (remove seeds if you don't like it hot)
A pinch of sea salt

1. Peel and chop the garlic and ginger and set aside (if you have more time, leaving garlic aside for 15 minutes at room temperature before cooking it can release more health-giving compounds). If you want to, now would also be a good time to roast your cashews in the oven, at 180°C/350°F/ gas mark 4 for 10 minutes. This is optional.

2. Add your noodles to boiling water with a pinch of salt and cook to packet instructions, drain and rinse them.

3. Chop up your spring onions, pak choi, mushrooms and chilli.

Continues opposite

For the sauce

2 tbsp sesame oil
1 tbsp maple syrup
4 tbsp soy sauce or
tamari
Juice of 1 ½ limes
Optional sprinkling
of sesame seeds
and cashew nuts,
to garnish

4. Add the sesame oil and heat on high. When it's piping hot, add your garlic and ginger, onions and chilli. After a couple of minutes, add the mushrooms and fry for a couple more minutes. If it starts to dry out, you can add a dash of apple cider vinegar.

5. Mix the juice of 1 ½ limes, the maple syrup and the soy sauce or tamari together in a small bowl.

6. Combine half of this sauce with your pak choi, cashews and peppers, and cook for another couple of minutes. You can leave a few cashews to one side to sprinkle on top.

7. Mix in the drained noodles and the rest of your sauce and cook for a couple more minutes.

8. Serve sprinkled with sesame seeds and the rest of the cashews.

Mushroom and Lentil Pie

. . . .

This is the definition of home-cooked and hearty food. My family love it. You can freeze leftover portions. I've added potato to the mash, as without it, the mash can be quite wet. I've used the chia seeds to thicken the sauce – as well as being nutritious, they absorb rather than dilute the flavours in the filling.

Makes 4 portions

You'll need: 25 x 20cm (10 x 8in) ovenproof casserole dish, a large saucepan and a potato masher

For the pie filling

10ml olive or rapeseed oil

1 large onion, finely chopped

3 cloves garlic, crushed

1 level tsp ground cumin

500g mushrooms, finely diced

1 red pepper, chopped

2 vegetable bouillon cubes or similar (some brands of beef stock cubes are meat-free and have a smoky flavour)

8 drops of liquid smoke (optional)

1 tbsp nutritional yeast

300ml water

Filling

1. In a large saucepan, add the oil and fry the onion until translucent. Add the garlic and cumin. Stir for 2 minutes, adding some splashes of water should the mixture stick.

2. Add the mushrooms. Stir and combine until they have reduced and released their liquid. Add the red pepper and continue to cook and stir.

3. After 5 minutes, add the water, stock cubes, liquid smoke and nutritional yeast. Cover and simmer for 10 minutes.

4. Add the lentils and simmer again for a further 5 minutes.

5. Stir in chia seeds to thicken. You may need more or less than the amount stated in the ingredients list. After a

Continues opposite

400g tin of green lentils, drained and thoroughly rinsed

1 tbsp milled chia seeds

Salt and pepper, to taste

For the mash topping

500g potatoes, peeled and chopped

700g root vegetables (combination of swede, carrot, squash, parsnip, etc.), peeled and chopped

20ml soy milk

Salt and pepper, to taste

1 sliced tomato, to garnish

10ml brush or spray of any oil

few minutes it should have a sauce-like consistency that you are happy with.

6. Add salt or pepper to taste.
7. Transfer to a pie dish and set aside to cool.

Topping

1. Preheat oven to 160°C/140°C fan/325°F/gas mark 3.
2. Peel and chop potatoes and root veg for boiling. Size the pieces in order of time they take to cook. Swede and carrot, for instance, will need to be cut smaller than parsnip and butternut squash. Boil and simmer until soft.
3. Drain the veg and then mash, adding any soy milk you feel you need to make the perfect mash. Add salt and pepper to taste.
4. Spoon mash evenly on top of filling.
5. Arrange sliced tomato and brush or squirt its top with the oil to help with browning.
6. Cook pie in the oven for 45 minutes, or until it's nicely browned on the top.

Katie's Charred Pepper and Garlic Pasta

. . . .

This is another lovely recipe from Katie, who shared her story on page 194. This oil-free pasta sauce requires only two steps and is packed with nutrition. Bold in flavour and luxuriously creamy, it's very simple to make!

Makes 4 portions

You'll need: a medium-depth saucepan, a hob and a blender or food processor

500g dried spaghetti (or other pasta, wholemeal optional)
4 large red peppers
8 garlic cloves
350g plain coconut yoghurt
5g nutritional yeast ('nooch')
1 red chilli
2 tsp salt
Juice of 1 lemon
1 handful fresh basil leaves
1 cup toasted nuts or seeds such as walnuts, almonds, sunflower or pumpkin seeds

1. Preheat oven to 200°C/400°F/gas mark 6.

2. Start by cooking some pasta of your choice in boiling water until al dente. Meanwhile, char the peppers by using metal tongs to place them directly onto a medium flame on your gas stovetop.

3. Turn the peppers around every few minutes until the skin is completely black. Alternatively, if you don't have a gas hob, halve them and lay them on a baking tray skin up in the oven for 20–30 minutes or until the skins are black. Then place the peppers in an airtight container for 10 minutes. This makes the skin easy to remove. Use a paper towel to rub off the skin, then remove the seeds and stalk.

4. Place them in a food processor or blender with the rest of the ingredients (except the fresh basil, nuts and seeds)

Continues opposite

plus 1 ladleful of the cooked pasta
water, and blitz until completely
smooth.

5. Transfer the sauce to a medium-
depth saucepan and simmer until the
colour darkens and it thickens slightly,
which takes about 10 minutes.

6. Meanwhile, toast the nuts or seeds in
a dry frying pan for 5 minutes on a
medium heat or in the oven at
180°C/160°C fan/350°F/gas mark 4
for 10 minutes, or until lightly
browned.

7. Now stir the sauce through the
spaghetti and serve with fresh basil
leaves and toasted nuts or seeds.

Cauliflower and Garlic Bechamel Spaghetti

· ·

Fancy a creamy pasta dish? Look no further! This is a super-simple Alfredo-style pasta that uses veggies instead of cream, milk and cheese. Packed with flavour and really easy to make, it will become a family favourite, I promise.

Makes 6 portions

You'll need: a baking tray, a saucepan, a food processor or blender and a sieve

1kg linguine
2 large bulbs/heads of garlic
2 medium cauliflowers
600ml oat milk
1 tsp Dijon mustard
4 tsp nutritional yeast (nooch)
10 sprigs thyme
6 sprigs rosemary
3 bay leaves
Fresh parsley or coriander, to garnish
Salt and pepper, to taste
Olive oil, to drizzle

1. Start by preheating the oven to 180°C/160°C fan/350°F/gas mark 4 and cut the cauliflower florets into pieces. Spread them out over a baking tray, drizzle with olive oil, salt and pepper. Put the garlic bulbs in some tin foil with olive oil, salt and pepper and wrap them. Add them to the same tray and put it in the oven and roast for 25 minutes.

2. Next, get a saucepan and add the oat milk with the thyme, rosemary, bay leaves and nooch and simmer over a low- or medium-heat hob for about 10 minutes so the flavours get into the milk. Then leave to cool. You can use a sieve to get the herbs out of the milk.

3. Start cooking the pasta; this usually takes around 8–10 minutes.

4. Get the cauliflower and garlic out of the oven. Add the cauliflower and

Continues opposite

garlic to a food processor (squeezing the garlic cloves out of their skins first) and, while it is still running, gently pour the sieved oat milk into the food processor and blitz the sauce until it is smooth.

5. Put the sauce in a pan and simmer gently, adding some of the cooked pasta water for extra creaminess. Taste and see if it needs more nooch, salt or pepper. Then drain the pasta and add it to the sauce in the pan, stir it together.

6. Chop up your fresh parsley or coriander and serve into pasta bowls immediately.

Dr Rupy Aujla's Story and Recipes

Dr Rupy Aujla is an NHS medical doctor whose life was suddenly changed when he suffered a significant heart condition called atrial fibrillation (AF) while working on the ward treating patients. Since learning more about nutritional medicine, he was able to reverse his condition using a food and lifestyle approach. In 2015 he started The Doctor's Kitchen on social media as a way of teaching everybody how they can cook their way to better health, and to showcase the beauty of food and the medicinal effects of eating and living well. His passion grew, and he created *The Doctor's Kitchen Podcast*, four bestselling cookbooks and now The Doctor's Kitchen app, as well as appearing regularly on the BBC, ITV and, more recently, alongside Prue Leith in Channel 4's *Cook Clever, Waste Less with Prue and Rupy*. Rupy says:

> Although I grew up with a strong foundation of under-standing the importance of food for nourishment, remembering my mother's chai and turmeric blends and the Ayurvedic traditions of healing from my grandparents, I rejected this wisdom in the early days of my medical career.
>
> But when I experienced a sudden and debilitating medical condition that required an intervention to burn an electrical pathway in my heart (an 'ablation'), my mother made me promise her that I'd try changes to my lifestyle before going under the knife. I agreed, and although I was sceptical, it made a difference. I began to centre my plate around plants, I started cooking for myself more often, I began prioritising proper exercise and 'downtime' in my life, and I even started a meditation practice.

What happened next surprised me as much as my specialists; my episodes of a racing and irregular heart rate diminished dramatically. Over a period of months, I realised I was coping without the use of medications, and that I had not required the ablation to fix my heart condition.

When I look back on this challenging time in my life, I am actually filled with gratitude. It allowed me to realise that teaching people how to cook their way to better health was just as much a part of my calling as working as an emergency medicine doctor was. It taught me that we need both modern medicine and holistic lifestyle changes to tackle chronic diseases.

One of the things that resonated most for me in Gemma's GLOVES framework was her focus on gratitude. For me, life is so much richer when I live it from a place of feeling thankful. Whatever life throws my way, if I consciously remember to focus on what I have rather than what I lack, I can start each day knowing how fortunate I am to be here, doing the things I do. Gratitude takes me back to my 'why'. It reminds me that my mission is based on helping others, just as healthy habits have helped me.

I chose these two recipes for this book because they are both super-easy creations that your taste buds, your budget and your body will all thank you for!

Dr Rupy's Pea and Sweet Potato Soup with Cardamom and Fennel

· ·

First up – the soup. The fusion of aromatic spices with sweet potatoes and fibre-rich peas is a beautiful combination that is very different from your average soup. Make sure you toast the spices – this really brings out the flavour.

Makes 4 portions

You'll need: a baking sheet, a large saucepan, a pestle and mortar or spice grinder and a stick blender

4 tbsp extra virgin olive oil

600g sweet potato, peeled and cut into 2cm cubes

4 tsp fennel seeds

2 tsp coriander seeds

8 cardamom pods, bashed

30g flat-leaf parsley, stalks and leaves chopped

400g frozen peas

200g frozen spinach

2 vegetable stock cubes, crumbled

40g pumpkin seeds, toasted and chopped

1.3l water

2 tbsp plant-based yoghurt (optional)

1. Preheat oven to 200°C/180°C fan/400°F/gas mark 6 and gather your ingredients.

2. Place the cubed sweet potato on a lined baking sheet. Drizzle with half of the oil and season before roasting for 25–30 minutes until soft.

3. In a large saucepan, dry toast the fennel seeds, coriander seeds and cardamom pods for 1 minute until fragrant. Take the spices off the heat and remove the seeds from the cardamom pods, before adding to a pestle and mortar. Pound all together until ground.

4. Return the spices to the saucepan along with the remainder of the oil and the chopped parsley stalks. Sauté for 2 minutes.

Continues opposite

5. Add the frozen peas, frozen spinach, roasted sweet potato, crumbled vegetable stock cubes and some salt and pepper. Stir together for 1 minute.

6. Add the water and simmer for 5–7 minutes before blending with a stick blender until smooth. Check the seasoning and serve with the parsley leaves and pumpkin seeds with a drizzle of oil and marbling of yoghurt.

Simple swaps

Sweet potato can be replaced with celeriac, parsnip or new potato.

Frozen peas can be switched for broad beans or edamame beans.

Frozen spinach can be replaced with chard or spring greens.

Dr Rupy's Black-eyed Pea Stew

My second recipe is an easy one-pot stew that will be great as a midweek meal, or to impress friends at dinner alongside some chunky toasted ciabatta or any grain or salad of your choice.

Makes 4 portions
You'll need: a casserole dish

2 tbsp oil of choice
2 medium white onions, sliced
2 medium red peppers, sliced
2 medium green peppers, sliced
2 tsp ground cumin
4 tsp paprika
1 tsp cayenne pepper
4 cloves garlic, grated
4 tomatoes, chopped
2 heaped tbsp tomato paste
2 x 400ml tin of coconut milk
2 x 400g tin of black-eyed peas, drained and thoroughly rinsed
300ml vegetable or mushroom stock
Juice of 2 limes
20g coriander, finely chopped

1. Heat the oil in a large-lidded casserole dish and add the onion and red and green peppers. Cook for 8 minutes, or until starting to soften.

2. Stir through the cumin, paprika, cayenne pepper and garlic and cook for a further 2 minutes.

3. Add the tomatoes, tomato paste, coconut milk, black-eyed peas, stock and a big pinch of salt and stir to combine. Bring to a simmer, then cover and cook for 15 minutes. Remove the lid for the last 5 minutes of cooking time.

4. Stir through the lime juice and coriander to serve.

Simple swaps

For red pepper/green pepper, you can use yellow pepper, courgette or leek.

For white onion, you can use red onion or leek.

For black-eyed peas, you can use borlotti beans, pinto beans or chickpeas.

Mexican Salad

· ′ · · · · ·

A hearty salad with beans, grains or vegetables can make a main meal, and in smaller portions can be used as a side dish, or in a picnic or lunchbox. As a general rule, make sure the grains and beans make up at least half of the dish, then the veg and leafy greens can make up about a quarter, and the dressings and nut/seed toppings about one-tenth of the salad. I love this Mexico-inspired salad; it tastes great on its own or as filling for a burrito.

The recipe calls for about half a large sweet potato, but you can roast the whole thing and use the rest for other dishes.

Makes 2 portions as a main, 4 as a side
You'll need: a large serving bowl, a baking tray and a saucepan

For the salad

100g sweet potato, cut into chunks
250g cooked brown rice (from a packet or cooked beforehand)
400g tin of black beans, drained and thoroughly rinsed
100g green beans
2 avocados, cut into chunks
50g cherry tomatoes, cut in half or quartered
1 bunch spring onions, thinly sliced
50g rocket leaves
1 handful fresh coriander, chopped

1. Cook the rice per the packet instructions. Preheat the oven to 180°C/160°C fan/350°F/gas mark 4 and chop the sweet potato into chunks, adding oil, salt and pepper.

2. Put the chunks in the oven on a baking tray for 25 minutes.

3. Bring some salted water to boil in a pan, add the green beans for 3 minutes or so, then immediately add them to very cold water to stop the cooking process and blanch them.

4. Chop the tomatoes, spring onions, avocados and coriander and put them to one side.

Continues overleaf

For the dressing

50ml olive oil

2 tbsp soy sauce or tamari

1 tbsp maple syrup

Juice of 2 limes

A pinch of salt

5. Mix all the ingredients for the dressing together and whisk with a fork. Drain and rinse the black beans.

6. Get a large serving bowl, add the brown rice in the bottom, then add the black beans, green beans, spring onions, tomatoes and avocados. Next drizzle over the dressing. Then add the sweet potato, rocket and fresh coriander and gently stir through. Serve and enjoy!

Gem-Gem Noodles

. . . .

My Australian cousin Freya first made this for me and claimed it was such a good recipe she had dreams about it. I wasn't sure whether to believe her, but after tasting it I can confirm it is indeed delicious – the stuff of culinary fantasies! I've enjoyed it many times since my return home. It's spicy, nutty and zingy and is adapted from 'Dan-Dan' noodles, a street food dish from Sichuan, China, and is named after the type of pole used by vendors to carry baskets of noodles across their shoulders. Freya called it 'Gem-Gem' in my honour and added tofu instead of pork!

Makes 4 portions

You'll need: a blender or a whisk to create the sauce, a saucepan and a wok/frying pan

For the noodles

1 tbsp vegetable or peanut oil

450g noodles (wheat, fresh or dried – glass or rice noodles for gluten-free option)

1 courgette, grated

2 celery sticks, finely diced

1 clove garlic, finely chopped

2 shallots, finely chopped

1 leek, chopped in half lengthways and finely chopped

1. Whisk together all the sauce ingredients with about a tablespoon of water.

2. Bring a saucepan of water with a pinch of salt to the boil and cook the noodles according to packet instructions. Rinse and set to one side.

3. Heat your wok or frying pan, add a tablespoon of oil and fry the leek and celery for about 2–3 minutes or until softened and smelling delicious.

4. Next, add the tofu, mushrooms and garlic, ideally covering each side of the tofu with oil as you fry it, until it is a golden colour. Mushrooms release

Continues overleaf

300g mushrooms, finely
    chopped (oyster,
    shitake, enoki or your
    favourite mushroom!)
200g medium or firm
    tofu, drained, patted
    dry and chopped into
    small cubes
Salt and pepper, to taste
1 tbsp white sesame
    seeds, toasted
1 bunch fresh coriander

For the sauce
2.5cm piece of fresh
    ginger, peeled and
    finely chopped
2 cloves garlic, finely
    chopped
2 tsp sugar (any kind)
2 tbsp soy sauce or
    tamari
2 tbsp rice vinegar
2 tbsp peanut oil (or an
    alternative like
    rapeseed or sunflower
    oil)
3 tbsp tahini (the runny
    kind)
1 tbsp water

juices, but after a few minutes, these should evaporate and they will also look golden.

5. Add the cooked noodles to the wok.

6. Pour the sauce on top of the noodles, and toss to combine.

7. Serve and top with the sesame seeds and fresh coriander. You can also drizzle chilli oil, if desired.

David Flynn's Story and Recipe

I confess it took me a long time to tell identical twins David and Stephen Flynn apart. David is one half of The Happy Pear – not only brothers, but also a lifestyle brand which now includes a café and sourdough bakery, an organic farm, six cookbooks, over 70 plant-based foods and a huge social media following.

The twins have also created genuine community around the concept of 'Swimrise' (getting up to swim with the rising sun) in their hometown of Greystones, Ireland. I've done Swimrise with David and Stephen, and (especially in February) it is a kind of cold that soaks right through to your bones in seconds. A refreshing dip in the Med it is not. And yet, there is something invigorating about it, and it speaks to one of the core tenets of the Happy Pear philosophy, and that is the creation of community. Spend any time with the Flynn brothers and it quickly becomes clear that what you see is what you get. They are positive people wanting to bring plant-based nutrition, meditation, yoga and community to the mainstream, and their life's mission shows no sign of slowing down. David says:

> We are identical twins, so we grew up competing for love and attention and as a result, we became overachievers. By the age of 21, we were playing semi-professional rugby, golf and modelling. We were studying business at the time as well, and money was what we were told would make us happy. We really didn't feel happy, despite following the path we thought we were supposed to. We felt

there must be more to life, and so we went travelling separately in 2001. Despite our physical distance from each other, we ended up both going vegan, giving up alcohol and getting super into yoga and community at the same time!

We wanted to share our newfound enthusiasm when we came home, and so we started The Happy Pear as a veg shop in 2004, aged 24, with a dream of creating a happier, healthier world and to inspire people to eat more veg! We must have seemed so idealistic at the time, and perhaps still do seem that way. But it was never just a veg shop to us; it was the centre of a revolution. A place where we could inspire others to build a healthy community around shared values of food that heals our bodies and the planet. The truth is that although we both tend to look on the bright side, I feel stress daily: when work piles up, the kids are pressing my buttons or too many things are coming at me at once.

What I love about Gemma's book is she doesn't just talk about how amazing food is for health. She mentions community, exercise and being in nature as well. For me, running, swimming, walking and yoga are so important to help me deal with stress. I like myself more when I do these things; I can breathe deeper, stand taller and just be more present. Nature also seems to take my problems from me. Swimming in the cold Irish Sea washes the stress off me, and gives me a fresh start every day.

I feel I know myself more now than I did when we started our business all those years ago – I accept myself more, I am better at saying no. Going for a walk with my wife by the sea fills my cup far more than the allure of fancy events and the opinions of others. Gemma's book reminds us that health is about so much more than food – living a connected life and appreciating nature are so important too.

David's 5-minute Daal Recipe

. . . .

The idea of cooking a curry in 5 minutes might seem a little far-fetched, but once you cook this, you will become a believer! It's a wonderful recipe to have in your repertoire as it's so tasty and easy to make, and you can easily adapt it to whatever ingredients you have in your kitchen.

Makes 6 portions

You'll need: a large pan and a toaster or grill

2 cloves garlic

2 thumb-size pieces fresh ginger

10 spring onions, chopped

400g tin of chopped tomatoes

2 x 400g tin of cooked chickpeas

2 x 400g tins of your preferred cooked lentils

100g baby spinach (approx. 2 handfuls)

2 x 400ml tin of coconut milk

Juice of 1 lime

1 large bunch of fresh coriander

1 tbsp any oil

20 cherry tomatoes

1. Drain and rinse the chickpeas and lentils. Peel and finely chop the garlic and ginger. Chop the spring onions and halve the cherry tomatoes. Pick the coriander leaves and finely chop the stalks.

2. Heat the oil on high heat in a large pan, non-stick if possible. Add the garlic and ginger to the pan, reduce the heat to medium and cook for 2 minutes, stirring occasionally.

3. Add the spring onions to the pan along with the cherry tomatoes, coriander stalks and salt. Cook for a further 1 minute.

4. Add the tins of chopped tomatoes, coconut milk, lentils and chickpeas, and stir well. Add in the spices, salt, black pepper and lime juice. Bring to a boil, then lower to a simmer for 5 minutes.

Continues opposite

1 tbsp curry powder
2 tsp salt
1 tsp black pepper
Wholemeal pitta
  breads, toasted to
  serve

5. Add in the spinach to wilt a few minutes before you serve, taste before serving and season if needed.

6. Serve with your toasted pittas and some fresh coriander and chilli flakes, if you like.

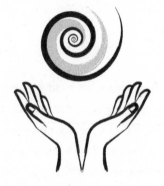

Exercise

I find that exercise is either the easiest or hardest healthy habit for my patients to integrate consistently. Exercise plans can bring up emotions of success, feeling powerful and accomplished or, for those who have struggled with body image, or who hated PE at school, the whole idea of exercising just dredges up bad memories. I hope the contents of this section can help to inspire even the most reluctant of you to move your bodies that little bit more because, as much as we want to avoid the truth:

We are made to move

Growing up, I was never one to exercise. Most kids run about a lot instinctively, and play is often the perfect way to begin a love for movement that lasts throughout our lives. But for me, an only child for a long time, books were my refuge. I was bigger than the other kids, more clunky and awkward. Always picked last for sports. Then puberty hit, and my sporting interest went from ambivalence to complete avoidance. My inactivity became a legacy that lasted for most of my life.

Overweight and with a high blood pressure, as a young doctor in training, I felt it was a 'now or never' moment, so I made the decision to buy some sportswear and finally get moving. I had learned how important exercise was from my medical training, and a couple of years into gruelling hospital shifts, I realised I needed to get fitter if I was going to cope with the schedule, long hours and emotional strain of my junior doctor years. That was one of the best decisions of my life, and it started me on a journey towards moving my body, culminating in completing the London Marathon in 2017 and 2021. Don't worry, I am not expecting you all to be marathon runners (unless you want to).

Along with our diets, being active is one of the main ways to achieve optimal health. And this does not just apply to physical fitness, but to our emotional wellness too. Whatever our starting point, the more we move our bodies throughout the day, the more this will benefit our health and wellbeing.

This is not about counting calories burned, but about helping our bodies to carry us comfortably through life.

Exercise makes you happier

A 2018 review of 23 studies, which altogether included 500,000 people, found that exercise was strongly linked to happiness, and that it didn't take much to have a benefit on our mood: just ten minutes a week![1] It can feel hard to get started, but in truth I don't know anyone without the time for ten minutes of exercise a week.

Other studies show that exercise has also been useful to treat active depression; a review of 25 randomised controlled trials found that exercise benefited both major and mild depression, and the benefits were even greater when participants exercised with other people.[2] This makes logical sense when we think about the connection and meaning we get from being with other people, and creating those social bonds around movement.

The type of exercise we do is not as important as the act of moving, although there have been studies showing that lifting weights can also boost your mood. A 2018 meta-analysis of 32 studies showed people doing resistance exercise consistently had fewer symptoms of depression, and it didn't matter if their training was only twice a week rather than every day – the benefits were the same.[3]

It can be so hard to motivate ourselves to move, and yet the feel-good factor once the work is done is hard to deny. The key seems to be in finding something you truly enjoy. If you haven't found that thing yet, don't worry. Trying something new is a great first step to discovering what works for you.

Exercise to live longer

Children tend to be able to concentrate more in school when they have been physically active – and the benefits of exercising young last well into our twilight years.[4] One study showed that when people had exercised regularly from the age of 15 to 25, they were able to process information faster between the ages of 62 to 85 years old.[5] The benefits of movement for prevention of dementia are crucial. Some studies show that the area of the brain responsible for storing memories – the hippocampus – can actually grow in response to exercise.[6,7]

Another study of 120 elderly people showed this hippocampal tissue growth in the brain was connected to being able to achieve better memory scores simply from walking for 40 minutes just 3 times a week for a year. The brains of the comparison group shrank over the course of the year.[8]

How could this happen?

Increased blood flow to the brain is a crucial benefit from moving our body, but exercise also helps neuronal growth and enhances connections between neurons by stimulating an important gene called the BDNF gene (brain-derived neurotrophic factor).[9] BDNF stimulates the growth and differentiation of neurons and synapses. It thrives in the areas of the brain that are important for learning and memory. BDNF can also be stimulated with laughter, sleep and intermittent fasting.[10,11,12]

You can slash your premature death risk by 20 to 30 per cent by walking 20 or 30 minutes a day compared to if you were to do no exercise at all.[13] Tens of thousands of women were followed in the Women's Health Study, and those who walked briskly for 60 to 90 minutes a week were found to have half the risk of a heart attack or a stroke. This was an observational study spanning over a decade.[14] But running for short periods may be even better; one study found that runners gained about three more years of life.[15] Just be careful with high-intensity exercise if you are new to it, especially if you have conditions that put you at risk, like high blood pressure or a previous heart attack. The key is to start slow and build up your fitness over time.

What about 10,000 steps a day? Could it be worth doing that much to ward off dementia? The 10,000 steps idea was created as part of a marketing campaign for an early pedometer device ahead of the Tokyo Olympic Games back in 1964. The Japanese character for 10,000 looks quite like a person walking, so the device was called the 'Manpo-kei', or 10,000 steps meter.[16] Interesting new research actually suggests that 10,000 steps is not far off an accurate estimate of benefits. A UK study from 2022 looking at nearly 80,000 adults between 40 and 79 years of age found that accruing more steps per day was associated with steady declines in dementia risk, up to 9,800 steps per day. Benefits did not increase past 10,000 steps. The 'dose' associated with 50 per cent of the benefits was 3,800 steps per day, and walking faster was associated with lower risk.[17] I'm just glad the Japanese character for 50 didn't look like a person walking; this is one marketing campaign which paid dividends for human health.

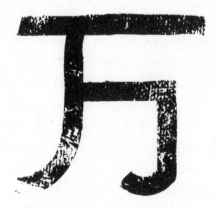

'Man', the Japanese symbol for the number 10,000.

Exercise keeps you young

Getting active is not only good for your lifespan, but also your youthfulness. Cellular ageing is slower when we move our bodies, as exercise can lengthen our telomeres. Telomeres are the little caps on the ends of our chromosomes, and the more our cells divide as they age, the shorter the telomeres become – until the cell dies. This is especially relevant when we are experiencing stress. One study showed exercise can have the power to lengthen telomeres that would otherwise have shortened from the stresses of being a caregiver to a loved one with dementia.[18]

In another study, adults who exercised a lot had a biological age nine years lower than their sedentary counterparts.[19] Your muscle size, reflexes, memories and immune system can all benefit from getting and staying active – and now is the perfect time to start.

Muscle mass begins to decline especially fast after the age of 65 – so the adage 'use it or lose it' has never been more relevant. Also studies show that resistance training (lifting weights or using your own body as resistance, like with a plank exercise) and endurance training (like running) can both increase bone density.[20] This is an important factor in reducing risk of osteoporosis and fractures later in life.

Making new muscle fibres doesn't just keep you strong, but it can also reduce your risk of dementia, improve your concentration and lift your mood.[21,22] This means bone strength is important, as well as balance, agility and resistance exercise. What could you do to get started if you're not used to movement? Walk between rooms of the house. Use tins of baked beans as mini-weights. Start a local walking group. Your body is a heavy weight, so you can use that if you don't want to buy dumbbells. If you have a garden, walk around it a few times a day. Gardening can become a new passion if it wasn't already! Look up a yoga class to try; it is never too late to improve balance and posture. Basically, do anything you can think of to keep those muscles moving, which will be vital to reducing risk of losing muscle mass and avoiding frailty.

Moving for your lymphatic system

In recent years it has been recognised that muscles are not just stretchy fibres that help us move – they are actually organs that produce their own proteins, like glands that secrete hormones. Incredibly, these muscle-made proteins, called cytokines, can signal between the muscles themselves and other, more distant organs in the body, to improve glucose uptake and breakdown of fats. This has a beneficial effect on our metabolism, improving weight control and potentially improving conditions such as type 2 diabetes.[23]

Why would *not* moving be so bad for us, irrespective of our weight? Your lymphatic system helps you get rid of dead cells, toxins and white blood cells that have worked hard to protect you from pathogens. Your lymph glands and organs include your tonsils, thymus and spleen. The lymph fluid your body makes has to be carried to nodes where it is cleaned before travelling to your neck veins and around the body. The trouble is, unless your muscles move, lymph fluid can become stagnant.

Your lymphatic system is entirely reliant on the contraction of your muscles to help lymph fluid move along. Deep breathing helps boost the pressure at the thoracic duct at the bottom of the neck to help lymphatic flow too – so the worst combination for your lymphatic system is stress and the shallow breathing that accompanies stress, coupled with lack of movement.

So when you feel your breathing is shallow and you have no motivation to move, a great first step to wake up your body is to breathe deeply, into your belly, and get that lymph fluid flowing. Then, you could try a 20-minute walk in the morning while breathing in the fresh air.

Move for vitality

So many young women get sold the 'bikini body' or 'hot girl summer' marketing lies. The truth is, there are so many great reasons to move that do not revolve around your beach body. As we have seen, you can do it for your 'old lady' body. Do it for your 'cancer-free' body.[24] If you don't want to think longer term, studies even show benefit for the prevention of gynaecological issues such as period pains, fibroids, endometriosis and PCOS.[25-28] Finally, exercise has also been shown to improve mood, confidence and self-belief. In a 2022 study of over 350 men and women, there was an association between exercising twice a week (compared to none) and higher levels of self-esteem, and an increased belief that participants could do the things they set out to do in life.[29] Movement really is a powerful elixir for mind and body.

Let's get started

Find a form of movement which is challenging enough that you could talk but not sing, and gradually increase from there. Guidelines vary but, in the UK, as a rule of thumb, the chief medical officer advises that preschoolers should spend at least 180 minutes (3 hours) per day physically active in some way, with children and young people between the ages of 5 and 18 having an hour a day of moderate- to high-intensity exercise.[30]

Adults are recommended to do a minimum of 150 minutes a week of moderate exercise – brisk walking or cycling counts as moderate exercise – or 75 minutes of more strenuous exercise, which includes running, sprinting or stair climbing. Guidelines also suggest including resistance exercises two days a week. How does this compare to what you do now?

Most of us do far less than this; it is good to understand what the recommendations are so we know how to optimise our routines and get on track with making movement work for us. If exercise is a struggle to fit into your day, see if the four-minute workout on page 246 helps, as well as the quick ideas at the end of this chapter.

How to breathe for better health

I want to take a moment to talk about an exercise our bodies do constantly, without us often thinking about it, if ever. We enter the world by taking a deep breath and then take somewhere between 17,000 to 30,000 breaths a day until we leave the world. Breathing is essential for life but also for the optimal functioning of mind and body.

Every relaxation technique in the world focuses on breathing and its ability to calm the mind and body. Even the most basic understanding of physiology helps to explain how breathing can affect the body.

Imagine a delicate set of scales, with the sympathetic nervous system on one side and parasympathetic nervous system on the other, working together in what's known as the autonomic nervous system (ANS). The ANS maintains normal bodily functions. When we are calm, we take slow and deep breaths, which engages the parasympathetic nervous system. This decreases heart rate and blood pressure, preparing the body for rest, sleep or digestion. Lovely.

The sympathetic nervous system prepares the body for physical or stressful situations by raising the heart rate, blood pressure, muscle tone and other functions, making us more alert and ready – sometimes this is called the fight-or-flight response. Fresh oxygen goes to the brain, glucose is shot into the body for energy, and faster breathing prepares your body for action.

The balance of these two systems can be delicate. If you feel stressed all the time, your sympathetic nervous system is more activated, which makes you constantly ready to react. If you come across a threat, such as 'a tree is going to fall on my head', this could be useful. But for dealing with being late for work, or making a mistake on a spreadsheet, being on high alert all the time exhausts your body.

Studies show that the sympathetic nervous system becomes overactive in cardiovascular diseases like chronic heart failure and hypertension.[31] It has also been associated with kidney disease, type 2 diabetes, obesity and even Parkinson's disease.[32-35]

The dysfunction of the sympathetic nervous system also underscores many mental health conditions, including anxiety and depression.[36] Irregular breathing, breathing through the mouth and chronic hyperventilation contributes to feelings of agitation and reduces oxygen to the brain.[37] Many people who have breathing difficulties will experience issues with anxiety. For example, anxiety is common in people who suffer from COPD (chronic obstructive pulmonary disease), one of our leading causes of death.[38]

The tricky thing is that the stimulation of both these systems is often completely unconscious. It is modulated through what we are doing, what and how we are eating, how we are sleeping, whether we exercise and even through our thoughts. Learning how to breathe consciously, and exercising consistently, are the two best ways to help keep your nervous systems in balance, making sure your sympathetic nervous system is not always on.

When we are feeling stressed, we tell ourselves or each other to 'take a deep breath'. In some ways this is counterintuitive, which I will explain, but there is actually a physiological reason behind this. While the responses of our ANS are completely outside of our conscious control, there is one exception to this: breathing.

The inhalation part of our breath engages the sympathetic nervous system, and the exhalation engages the parasympathetic nervous system. When we slow our breathing and focus on extending the exhalation, our lungs and heart can 'feed back' to our brain and tell it that we are calm and peaceful, even if we are feeling stressed. If we keep our exhalation longer than our inhalation for a few minutes, the respiratory cycle will slow down our heart rate, shifting the balance further towards the parasympathetic nervous system. It engages our vagus nerve, the long and winding cranial nerve that extends from our brain to our gut, linking the heart, lungs and digestive system. This is a neural decelerator and slows the entire system, telling it to relax.

So why is it a problem when we just 'take a deep breath'? Because when we are trying to fill lungs that are already half full of air, we feel more constricted in our breath. Pushing all the air out of our lungs first is far more helpful, because then the air can slowly relax back into the body, with a focus on the belly – not the chest. Doing this will help to slow and regulate your rhythm of breathing and will naturally extend your exhalation. This helps engage your parasympathetic nervous system.

The truth is that many people breathe too quickly, and take shallow breaths, which alters the natural levels of gases in the blood. This reduces the amount of oxygen that gets to tissues and causes constriction of the smooth muscles surrounding blood vessels and airways. By bringing breathing volume towards normal and making the switch from mouth to nose breathing, we help to improve health issues such as hay fever, asthma and sleep apnoea. [39-42] Breathing through the nose also helps to filter and moisten the air. This protects the airways from pathogens (nose hairs *are* useful!) and avoids drying out your gums and the tissue lining the inside of your mouth. Nose breathing maintains natural bacteria, which can help prevent gum disease and tooth decay as well. [43] Amazingly, the paranasal sinuses continually produce nitric oxide (NO), an incredible gas that diffuses to the bronchi and lungs to open up the airways and the blood vessels. [44] Studies indicate that NO may also help to reduce respiratory tract infections by inactivating viruses. [45] So remember – the mouth is for eating and talking, and the nose is for breathing.

There are various breathing techniques that focus on slowing breath and/or extending the exhalation. Just choose the one that you find easiest to fit into your day. I would also add some emphasis here on breathing through the nose rather than the mouth for these exercises. This is because nose breathing stimulates the diaphragm, which is directly connected to the vagus nerve, helping us to breathe more efficiently. [46] Breathing techniques can also use the power of holding breath. When we hold our breath, nitric oxide can build up in the nasal cavity. This is a good thing because, as mentioned, NO can help our blood vessels relax. Enzymes that make this important gas are present in the nose and in the sinuses around the nose. By holding the breath and then breathing in through our noses, we allow this gas into our lungs far more efficiently.

I remember my patient Louise, who had a long history of obsessive-compulsive disorder and generalised anxiety disorder. This has impacted her in a number of ways, and more recently had stopped her from feeling able to leave the house. The amount of different checks she felt she needed to do before leaving (a set ritual of checking all the windows and doors, washing her hands and repeating the window and door checks a series of five times) simultaneously eased her anxiety (as she was beginning the rituals) and heightened it (when she realised she was nearing the time she had to leave and she would potentially be late for work).

In combination with therapy and medication, I also offered her the opportunity to try the 4-7-8 breathing technique (see page 242) when she could feel her anxiety rising, or if her ritual was interrupted in some way and she wanted to start it again. We practised it together. The next time I saw her, she told me she had had a great breakthrough. In doing the breathing technique before she got out of bed each morning, she had been able to play a game with herself to reduce the rituals from five times to four. She felt okay. So the next week she had reduced her ritual to three repetitions, then two and then one. By the time I saw her again in clinic, she had kept it to once and was able to regulate her breathing when she felt the strong urge to start the cycle again. It was an incredible win, as it meant her quality of life improved dramatically – she was able to leave the house in good time and felt a lot less anxiety when out of the house as well. A wonderful win for the power of the breath!

How to breathe well

I don't like the word 'mindfulness' because, to me, an *emptier* mind, or at least the ability to allow ourselves a certain distance from our thoughts, is really valuable. We can't really stop our steady stream of thoughts and, contrary to popular belief, stopping our racing mind is not the purpose of mindfulness, or even of meditation. Instead, it's about being more aware of our current emotions, sensations and surroundings. It is about awareness. But what does it mean to 'be aware'?

Simply becoming aware of our thoughts, and maybe even visualising them as being on the floor, or at arm's-length from us, rather than inside our head, is a simple way to remind us that we are not our thoughts. There are lots of ideas and judgements that come into our minds uninvited, usually as a result of the external world, or the pressures we feel.

Awareness can start simply in the act of creating a conscious distance between us and our thoughts. We can begin to notice that we are the person watching those thoughts roll by, rather than the thoughts themselves. One of the most powerful ways to involve our bodies in the process of helping us do this is to engage the breath.

1. Always start with pushing air out of your lungs. When they feel empty, make a 'shhhh' sound to empty them a bit more. When you push all the air out of your chest first, on your next in-breath, you are replenishing lungs that are not already half full.

2. Extend your out-breath longer than your in-breath. If you like 'box breathing' (see opposite) and you want to make the out-breath longer, you can visualise a rectangle, rather than a square.

3. Aim to breathe in through your nose, if you can.

Breathing for stress – or a concentration boost

Known as 'box breathing or 'square breathing', this is a visualisation exercise that encourages us to take slow and deep breaths. People with chronic obstructive pulmonary disease (COPD) might find it particularly beneficial.[47] If you get dizzy after a few rounds, stay sitting for a few minutes and resume the exercise. If you do this several times a day, you will soon get used to it and find it a beneficial tool to use when you are feeling stressed, or are in need of a concentration boost.

❈ Make sure you are sitting upright in a comfortable chair with your feet flat on the floor – keep your hands in your lap and your posture relaxed.

❈ Slowly exhale, getting all the oxygen out of your lungs for four seconds.

❈ Hold your breath for a slow count of four seconds.

❈ Slowly inhale for four seconds, completely filling your lungs.

❈ Hold your breath for a slow count of four seconds.

❈ Exhale for four slow counts.

❈ Repeat the cycle four times.

❈ Imagine a square as you do this exercise – each equal side is an out-breath, hold, or in-breath for the count of four.

Relaxing breathing – for anxiety and insomnia

This is the 4-7-8 breathing that helped my patient Louise, and it has roots in yoga's pranayama. It is slightly harder to master than box breathing, but has been described by its creator Dr Andrew Weil as a 'natural tranquilliser for the nervous system'. It can be particularly useful if you are suffering from insomnia.[48] Remember to focus your breath on the stomach area; abdominal breathing with our bellies can help manage many conditions, including anxiety, insomnia, depression, high blood pressure and COPD.[49]

* Make sure you are comfortably sitting upright with your feet flat on the floor – keep your hands in your lap and your posture relaxed.
* First exhale completely through your mouth, making a whooshing noise.
* Inhale slowly through your nose for a slow count of four seconds.
* Hold your breath for a count of seven seconds.
* Exhale through your mouth for a count of eight seconds. This is one cycle.
* Repeat the cycle three times.

One-minute reset

This is a simple tip I first learned about from fellow GP Dr Ayan Panja.[50] Does one minute of your time have the power to change your whole day? I believe so, yes. Engaging your parasympathetic nervous system (by breathing out for longer than you breathe in) for just one minute can reset your state of mind and bring you back to who you want to be.

Use one of the breathing techniques on the previous pages, in combination with visualising your favourite relaxing place, perhaps a forest or a beach, or someone you love. I have found a one-minute reset is particularly useful during transitions in my day, like driving home from work, before picking my kids up from school, or after a difficult meeting or consultation and before 'the next thing'. It is a one-minute reminder that the rest of your day does not have to be defined by what came before it. Could you fit the one-minute reset into your routine?

Breathe and laugh

Deep and slow breathing helps stimulate the vagus nerve and activate the calming parasympathetic nervous system in the same way that laughter does.[51] Being the kind of person who laughs easily really is good for you, and for those that you love. Remember laughing is not just for the good times – studies show that laughter can help us accept and move through tough times too.[52,53] Many medics know this and often bond through dark humour. Finding the ridiculous when life gets tough can be a way of bonding and easing the stress and tension we feel. There is even such a thing as 'laughing yoga', and forced laughing (which soon turns into real laughter!) is recommended as part of the Chinese art of self-healing (known as 'Yang Sheng', or 'nourishing life'). Like yoga, Yang Sheng is an ancient wellness practice.[54,55] Why not try a simple round of ten slow, deep breaths (start with the out-breath) three times daily and see how you feel? Or find some funny videos on YouTube to get you started!

Shake it off

Have you ever seen a dog shake themselves off after having jumped in water? A large dog can shake 70 per cent of the water off his fur in just four seconds. In fact, all mammals do this as a way to protect against hypothermia, from mice to kangaroos! Incredibly, a full-body shake can generate centrifugal forces 10 to 70 times that of gravity.[56]

There is another important reason a mammal will do the full-body shake – to relieve tension. Wild animals naturally and instinctively release adrenaline and cortisol by doing a full-body shake. It can happen after a chase between a lion and a deer (both mammals will do this) and in domesticated animals, it can happen after a shock or an excitement. My dog Rosie gives a full-body shake after she greets me, once the initial excitement of saying hello subsides. Once the shake is done, excess energy has been released. Then the animal can simply carry on, and do what animals do.

The thing is, we are also mammals. Rather than storing stress, one simple way to release it is to have a physiological shake, or to induce a tremor response in the muscles with some simple stretches. The full-body shake is one of the emotional-release strategies in Yang Sheng. It is described as a way of processing emotions: by recognising them, then allowing them to move physically through the body as a way to release them. This might be done in various ways, including laughter, singing, dancing or shaking. Shaking is also a part of yoga practices (in the form of psoas muscle hip-opener stretches that can induce tremor as well as active shaking movements). There is a type of physical therapy that has become popular as an extension of these ancient practices; it's called 'tension release exercises' and aims to do exactly that. For simple stress relief, these stretches can be done at home. But if you are diagnosed with PTSD or another mental illness that means releasing emotions makes you more vulnerable, it's advised to do them with a trained practitioner.[57]

The shake

This is a simple energy shifter when nervous, excited or just hoping to wake yourself up or shift a negative thought spiral. If you want to see the shake in action, I thoroughly recommend you follow Chinese medicine practitioner Katie Brindle on social media. To know more about Yang Sheng practices such as qigong, you can read her book *Yang Sheng: The Art of Chinese Self-Healing* as an introduction to this ancient practice.

1. While standing, shake both arms at the same time, releasing all tension and imagining they are like jelly.
2. While still shaking your arms, lift and shake your left leg, then your right.
3. Then, add in a shake of the head left to right (you can smile while doing this!).
4. Next, you can add in a wrist and forearm shake on both sides.
5. Now shake your hips, your shoulders and whole body, turning it into a shimmy or a shake, if that feels good.
6. As an added extra, you can channel your favourite dance moves – whether that's Elvis's pelvis thrusting and leg shaking, The Beatles ('Twist and Shout'), Taylor Swift ('Shake It Off') or City Girls and Cardi B ('Twerk'). Let it all go and have fun!

The four-minute anytime, anywhere workout

This is a quick workout for everyone, and it can fit into even the busiest of schedules. It takes four minutes and works all your major muscle groups. The simple bursts of movement are easy to remember. No special equipment is needed, just you and your body.

The workout consists of four sets of repetitions of the following exercises.

There are just four things to remember.

Squats

Find a foot stance that works for you, with your feet hip-width apart and your feet forwards. Tense your abs and stand tall. Sit

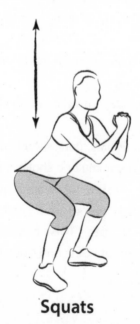

Squats

down into the squat, moving your bottom backwards, and shift your weight onto your heels. As you descend, push your knees slightly outwards; your knees should be directly above your toes. Push your arms up, pointing straight out in front of you, for balance. Look ahead and keep your back straight. Rise back up, driving up through your heels.

Circular arm swings

Stand with your feet hip-width apart and your arms beside your thighs. With your fists tight, raise both arms over your head, as if you are making a rainbow shape, touching your hands at the top and bottom of the motion. If you have a shoulder injury, start with

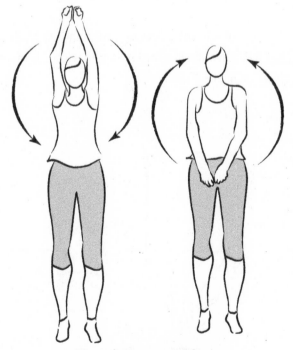

Circular arm swings

your hands in a prayer position in front of your chest and make circular motions round and towards the centre of your chest, as if you are doing breaststroke. You can progress to controlled star jumps if/when you feel able to.

Tricep dips

Sit on the edge of a stable chair or a sofa and grip the edge next to your hips. Your fingers should be pointed at your feet, your legs extended and your feet about hip-width apart, with the heels touching the ground. To make it easier, you can bend your knees and have your feet flat on the floor. Look straight ahead with your chin up. Remember to keep your shoulders down, away from your ears.

1. Press down into the palms of your hands to lift your body and slide forward just far enough that your bottom clears the edge of the chair.

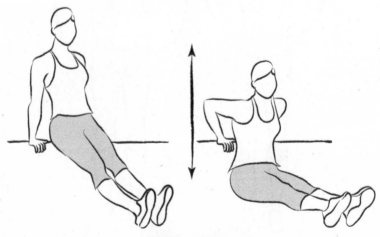

Tricep dips

2. Lower yourself until your elbows are bent between 45 and 90 degrees. Control the movement throughout the range of motion.

3. Push yourself back up slowly until your arms are almost straight, and repeat (don't lock your elbows).

If tricep dips are challenging . . .

From a standing position, lean forward at the waist with a straight back and a slight bend in your knees. Let your arms hang loose, then bend your elbows and keep your arms tight to your sides as you bring your elbows up, so your shoulder blades touch. Make your movements controlled. When you're ready, you can hold some tins of beans or water bottles in your hands to add resistance.

Arm raises

Stand with your feet shoulder-width apart. Keep your arms straight and raise each arm alternately in front of you, so they are at a 90-degree angle to your body, in a controlled swinging motion. Keep your arms tight and your muscles engaged, and avoiding swinging your arms too high or low. (See the illustration on the next page.)

If you aim for ten repetitions of each exercise, this takes about four minutes. If you wish, you can build up the repetitions as your fitness increases. You don't need any equipment or to lie down; there are no trainers or sportswear. Just you and your body. Anytime, anywhere.

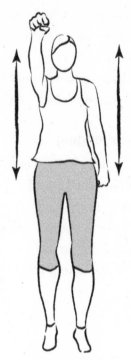

Arm raises

Starting the day with a morning stretch

A morning stretch will make you feel more awake and ready to start your plant-powered day! Stay in each position for five deep breaths to further engage your parasympathetic nervous system. For each out-breath, see if you can stretch the position a little bit further . . .

1. Lie on your back and reach your arms up over your head – breathe.
2. Slowly bend your knees so your feet are flat on the floor.
3. Move your knees over to the left – breathe.

4. Move your knees over to the right – breathe.

5. Move your left foot over your right knee and bring your arms through the space this creates to hug the back of your right thigh into your chest – breathe. Move your left foot back.

6. Swing your right foot over your left knee and repeat the hug. Breathe. Remember to sink deeper into the stretch gently with each out-breath.

7. Return to a neutral position, with your knees bent and your arms relaxed by your sides, and gently rest your knees out on either side like a frog, keeping your feet together. Take your final five deep breaths.

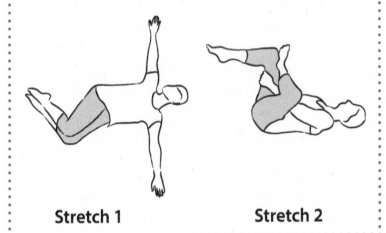

Stretch 1   **Stretch 2**

How to keep moving

Under pressure, we tend to fall back on old comforts. New habits rarely stick unless we attach them to old habits, like doing jumping jacks while making a cup of tea, or a few quick press-ups before jumping in the shower. Remember our talk about values shaping identity on page 94? If we say we are a 'couch potato' or that 'I've never been able to exercise', then the new habits to move your body won't stick. So it's time to put a stake in the ground.

Ideas to try

- ❋ As soon as you wake up, can you move your body?
- ❋ Wearing workout clothes to bed is one easy step to encourage you to move your body as soon as you wake up. No getting cold and getting changed – all you have to do is get moving.
- ❋ Sign up for an event you will run for a charity you like and tell people 'I'm into running now'.
- ❋ Follow new mentors on social media, so that you can see your lifestyle choice reminders when you go online. Remember to choose accounts that inspire you, not ones that make you feel bad!
- ❋ As you wait for the kettle to boil to make a cup of tea, could you do some sit-ups?
- ❋ As soon as you have picked up the kids from school, could you dance around the kitchen together?
- ❋ Just before lunch and just before dinner are convenient times to get moving without indigestion or too much thought.

What has been your favourite movement tip from this chapter? Make a note of it in the journal pages at the back of the book and you can incorporate it into your very own *Get Well, Stay Well* plan later on in the book.

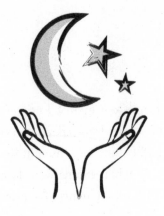

Sleep

I used to think sleep was a luxury. I cringe now when I think of all the years where I stayed up too late, didn't bother going to bed after night shifts and thought sleeping was a waste of precious study time when exams were looming. But sleep is one of the most important elements of ensuring good health in the long term.

Sleep deprivation has now reached epidemic levels.[1] Why? Our social lives and work have changed so much. Computers, tablets and smartphones keep us awake. We lead more sedentary and indoor lives. Working days can bleed more easily into home life because of technology that allows us to always be 'on'. And we are influenced by social pressures that encourage the view that being busy is a badge of honour, and that sleeping is equated with laziness.

If you feel this way, let's consider ways to change your mind. Sleep is vital – just as exercise and a good diet help us stay well, sleep can also help us maintain our weight and ward off serious problems like heart attacks, obesity, cancer and Alzheimer's disease.[2-5]

One in three of us suffers from poor sleep, and in some groups, such as children, experts describe sleep issues as 'a hidden health crisis', with vast numbers of families accessing hospital treatment for sleep disorders and ADHD, which is associated with difficulty 'switching off' and getting to sleep.[6] I see so many patients suffering from insomnia. These patients also often have depression and anxiety, which is fuelled by their inability to switch off and sleep.[7] If you have struggled with insomnia, the good news is there are ways you can improve your sleep through lifestyle. You may feel like you have tried everything, from lavender on the pillow to a strict sleep routine and calming chamomile tea. Don't worry – there are plenty of ideas scattered throughout this chapter, and within each of the other parts of the GLOVES framework too. These tips will help restore healthy sleep as well as other areas of your general wellbeing. If you are still struggling, I suggest you seek the support of a specialist sleep clinic, which can help you learn a series of techniques for better sleep that are based on cognitive behavioural therapy. This is known as CBT-i.[8]

But first, let's understand why it is worth prioritising good sleep, if you don't already. There are so many reasons why sleep is good for you. These include:

- ❀ **Better mood.** Sleep allows you to process your emotions more effectively and develop a more positive outlook. Chronic lack of sleep puts you at greater risk of developing mental health issues, such as depression and anxiety.[9] In fact, brain scans reveal the amygdala, a key spot in the brain for triggering anger, is 60 per cent more reactive in those who are sleep deprived.[10]

- ❀ **Healthier heart.** Lack of sleep is also linked to coronary heart disease, no matter your age, weight, exercise levels or if you smoke.[11,12] It is thought that around six to eight hours of sleep per night is the optimal level for a healthy heart. Although the links between heart health and sleep are not crystal clear, disturbed sleep is linked to higher levels of a protein called CRP, which is a sign of inflammation.[13]

- ❀ **Easier to maintain a healthier weight.** Have you ever found that when you've had a bad night's sleep you reach for a sugary snack? Research shows that being sleep deprived alters the levels of two hormones linked to appetite and satiety – ghrelin and leptin.[14] Poor sleep is consistently linked to weight gain and obesity. A meta-analysis of studies found that short sleep duration increased the likelihood of obesity by 89 per cent in children and 55 per cent in adults.[15] Our cells also become less sensitive to insulin, which means we will also be more prone to diabetes.[16,17] If you are aiming for a healthy body weight, good sleep is a priority.

❀ **Stronger immune system.** Sleep allows your body to rest and repair. Research shows that sleep improves immune cells known as T-cells, white blood cells that are critical to the body's immune response.[18] One study showed that sleep improves the potential ability of some of the body's immune cells to attach to their targets, explaining why sleep can help to fight off infection.[19]

❀ **Improved concentration and attention.** Consistent sleep patterns have been linked to children performing better at school.[20] Good sleep helps us to think more clearly, make decisions, and remember more.[21] When we sleep, connections between brain cells are strengthened and information is stored as long-term memories, making it easier to recall information.[22] Sleep also feeds creativity and innovative thinking.[23]

❀ **You are much safer.** Your reaction times are much slower when you have not had enough sleep, and in tests, sleep-deprived drivers perform in a similar way to drunk drivers.[24] With five hours of sleep or less, your chances of being in an accident are much higher.[25]

❀ **Natural painkiller.** When we sleep better, research shows we are able to tolerate pain better.[26,27] For chronic pain sufferers this can be very difficult, as pain leads to lack of sleep and it can become an ongoing problem. There is research that shows that not getting enough sleep can interfere with the mechanisms of some pain-relieving drugs.[28]

✻ **Reduced Alzheimer's risk.** Amyloid is a protein that is found in our brains and bodies, but in Alzheimer's disease, amyloid sticks together and forms clumps that later become plaque in the brain. The amyloid deposits that accumulate in the brains of people with Alzheimer's dementia are cleaned away during sleep.[29] Without sleep, toxic metabolites can build up, attacking and degrading the brain's deep-sleep-generating regions. It then becomes a vicious cycle. If you or a loved one has memory issues, my sleep tips will be really valuable in improving your memory and functioning in the years to come.[30]

The bottom line is this: the shorter your sleep, the shorter your life. If you make time for movement, make time for sleep too – it is free, widely available and is guaranteed to extend the quality and length of your life.

There are no hard and fast rules when it comes to exactly the right amount of sleep for every individual – the key thing is not to overlook your sleep experience when you are not feeling well, and not to think you can power through life without prioritising sleep.[31] The hours of total sleep that we need over a 24-hour period varies over our lifetimes. On average, adults need around 7 to 8 hours of sleep per night, but children need much more. Babies typically sleep for around 16 hours per day, young children need 10 to 11 hours a night, and teenagers need around 9 or 10 hours.

Don't lie in

We cannot make up for sleep deprivation. Although we think that having a lie-in on a weekend will temporarily improve things, it will not make up for our overall 'sleep debt'.[32] Sleep debt is the amount of time we should be asleep versus the amount of time we do sleep. In fact, circadian rhythm (day–night rhythm) disruptions happen when we wake early on a weekday and lie in on a weekend. Interestingly, research has found the most common day of the week to be admitted to hospital with a serious heart attack is Monday.[33] We know heart attacks and strokes are more likely to happen in winter and in the early hours of the morning.[34,35] Previous studies have also shown a higher rate of heart attacks in the days following the clocks going forward for daylight savings time.[36] The authors of the most recent study on this believe this phenomenon is caused by the circadian rhythm affecting circulating hormones that can influence heart attacks and strokes.[37] The best way to help yourself in this regard (as well as avoiding stress) is to establish a healthy sleep routine.

Do not feel guilty or silly for choosing to have an early night to enable you to sleep for longer. We may think of sleep as a time when our bodies and minds 'shut down', but this is not the case: sleep is a time where our brains and bodies are active. Our brains are processing experiences and memories, where short-term memories are filed in a process called 'consolidation'. Our bodies also need sleep to restore and rejuvenate muscles and tissues, and to synthesise hormones. It has also been found that sleep plays a 'housekeeping' role, removing toxins from our brains.[38] The astroglial cells (a type of brain cell) form a network of channels next to the blood vessels inside the brain. These channels allow the smooth flow of cerebrospinal fluid (the fluid that coats and protects our brains) and works as a type of waste-disposal system.[39] It's called the glymphatic system. Just as the lymphatic system transports lymph fluid, and the cardiovascular system transports blood, so the glymphatic system transports toxic metabolites out of the fluid surrounding the brain. While this can happen when we are awake, it has been found that clearance of toxins is much faster when we are asleep.[40] Let your body get busy doing essential health repairs while you snooze.

The full function of sleep is still a mystery to us at the time of going to press, but while scientists do more research, what we know now is that sleep affects every organ and tissue in the body, and that chronic lack of sleep increases the risk of serious disease, including heart disease, depression, obesity and diabetes.[41,42] Being awake for 17 hours makes us as impaired as if we were drunk.[24] And just one night of four or five hours of sleep means our natural killer cells (white blood cells that destroy infected cells and cancer cells in your body) will fall by around 70 per cent.[43] Lack of sleep is also associated with bowel, breast and prostate cancer.[44-46]

What happens while we sleep?

Throughout your time asleep, your brain repeats two processes: REM (rapid eye movement) sleep and non-REM sleep. Both are exactly as they sound: in REM sleep, your eyes move rapidly under your eyelids, and in non-REM sleep, your eyes are still. Each is linked to specific brain activity. During non-REM sleep, our bodies relax, blood pressure drops and the brain becomes less sensitive to external stimuli, so we are less likely to wake up. It is during this phase that our bodies repair and renew.[47]

During REM sleep, when we dream, our brains reorganise

information and make memories, clearing out irrelevant information and storing other information, boosting memory and neural growth. During this phase, our body temperature and heart rate increases and our blood pressure rises.[48]

Together, these two types of sleep make one complete sleep cycle, which takes around 90 minutes.[49] Your body cycles through this ideally around four or five times a night. The ratio of non-REM to REM sleep changes throughout the night, with non-REM sleep dominating the first part of the night and REM kicking in later on. This is why many sleep scientists say the sleep we get before midnight is the most important.[50]

Everyone's sleep pattern is individual and depends on our daily experiences, which all impact the hormones that enable us to sleep. Remember the crucial role vitamin D, serotonin and melatonin play in sleep (see pages 108–9)? Some of the factors at play are:

* ❋ how we feel – including stress
* ❋ what we eat and drink
* ❋ how active we are

Our genetics play a role and there is also normal biological variation. A small proportion of us suffer with delayed sleep phase disorder (DSPD), which typically delays our cue to sleep by about two hours.[51] This is thought to be a mutation in the CRY1 gene, which would perhaps have been useful to early humans in that one of the tribe could stay up later and look out for danger to the group – but not so useful when one of the biggest risks to health in the modern age is insomnia.

Most of us, despite instinctively classing ourselves as either 'morning larks' or 'night owls', are more impacted by artificial light.[52,53] It's our devices and our caffeine-fuelled lifestyles that keep us staying up later than our biological clock would dictate.

Questions to help you determine the quality of your sleep

Below are a few questions you can ask yourself to assess the quality of your sleep. If you tend to answer 'often' or 'almost always' to these questions, you'll benefit the most from the tools in this chapter.

- Do you tend to feel groggy when you wake up?
- Do you find it hard to get going without your morning coffee?
- Do you have trouble falling asleep?
- When you wake in the night, is it hard to get back to sleep?
- Do you have a medical condition that wakes you from sleep?
- Do you tend to breathe through your mouth?
- Does your partner tell you that you snore?
- Do you make mistakes at work because you are tired?
- Do you feel forgetful because you are tired?
- Are you irritable due to tiredness?
- Do you have appetite changes due to tiredness?

If any of these are questions you relate to, read on for some tips that may improve your sleep, and your quality of life.

Advice for shift workers

I see many shift workers in my clinics. These are the nurses, para-medics, firefighters, factory workers, HGV drivers, commercial cleaning staff and others who keep our countries running and who work outside of the nine-to-five working day that most people follow.

Society keeps running because of the sleep sacrifices these people make. I experienced how hard shift work can be on our bodies earlier in my career when I was doing 24-hour shifts and regular rotas with a week of night shifts as part of them. I was so lucky not to be sitting exams at that time or trying to look after kids or other loved ones while having to navigate night shifts, as so many others have to.

Sometimes people do not mention their sleep patterns when they come to see me, so unless I ask them, it can be hard to make the correlation between their health issues and their sleep patterns, but we know that lack of sleep is linked to certain chronic diseases, as well as decreased performance and productivity.

It is so important for people who work shifts to be aware of this and regulate their sleep cycles wherever possible. Here are some strategies to follow to ensure good rest:

* **Set aside seven to nine hours to sleep.** Where possible, ensure you have a solid window of time in which to sleep and make sure that friends and family know not to disturb you in that time. Pop a note on the fridge for your family, or a notice on the front door to warn any delivery drivers. When you have finished your shift, do not be tempted to delay going to bed – I

know only too well the feeling of desperation for some 'me' time, a chance to unwind, watch TV or run some errands. The problem is that this will make you feel more alert and delay your sleep further. Go to bed as quickly as possible.

❀ **Follow a routine.** Follow the same routine to prepare for sleep, whatever the time of day or night. This will encourage your body to recognise a pattern and signal that it is time for rest. So take a bath, listen to music or do some simple breathing exercises as part of your wind-down routine. See the 'How to breathe well' section on page 240 for details.

❀ **Create a restful environment.** Keep technology out of your bedroom and use blackout curtains or an eye mask to ensure the room is as dark as possible. This will be essential for daytime sleepers. If you live in a noisy environment, ear plugs will help too. If you see yourself working shifts for many years, you could decide to invest in soundproofing measures, such as double glazing, heavy curtains, wall insulation and thicker carpets.

❀ **Recover between shifts.** Where possible, try to find time for recovery between shifts. Regular exercise will help you stay physically fit and less fatigued. Short naps of less than half an hour before your shift may also help you feel more alert.

❀ **Use light.** Daylight is a signal to the body to stay awake, so use dark glasses as you come home from a shift and turn all the lights down – make your space as dark as possible to encourage your body to produce melatonin. Seek out natural light or use artificial bright light only before and in the early part of your shift.

❋ **Eat well.** In my experience, many shift workers suffer from digestive issues and can have a tendency to skip meals, eat irregularly or eat unhealthy foods. It is important to think about the timings and quality of your meals. Have healthy foods available at home and prepare meals where possible, so they are ready to eat when you get home from your shift. Eat small, frequent meals rather than large, heavy ones and choose foods that are easy to digest, like salads and soup (see pages 190–225 for inspiration). Ensure you are well hydrated. Try not to drink any caffeine when you think you need it most – within the four hours at the end of your shift. You'll regret it when you're staring at the ceiling counting sheep . . .

My patient Joe worked as a night porter at the local hospital and relied on Mars Bars and cups of coffee to keep him going throughout his long night shifts. When he came to see me, he was struggling terribly with headaches and exhaustion. He wanted to get some sleeping tablets to help him rest during the day so he could continue with his rota. He could not afford to take time off work, and he had three night shifts left before returning to days again. He found the on-and-off day shift–night shift schedule really affected his mood, and he would snap at his kids, when he was waking up from his daytime sleep, for being too loud as he slept, and sometimes Joe felt so fed up that days would go by without him smiling, playing with his kids or finding anything worth getting excited about. We talked about how long this pattern had been going on (coming up to a year), and we decided to tackle it head-on, rather than relying on sleeping tablets, caffeine and sugar.

What worked for Joe? He chose to prepare overnight oats each day with berries, nuts and seeds that he could take into work and use as a snack when he was feeling hungry. He took a big bottle of flavoured water into work instead of the huge coffee flask he was used to, and decided one coffee at the start of his shift would be his limit before starting on the flavoured water. Joe also decided to wear his sunglasses on the way home from his shift, and make an effort to notice the bright artificial lights early on in his shift to try and set his sleep–wake cycle like the early morning light would. He also invested in blackout blinds for his bedroom, a low-light bedside table lamp to help create a relaxing environment, and silicone earplugs with an eye mask to wear when he slept – all with the intention to reduce the chances he would wake up too early or be disturbed by noise in the house.

After a month he returned for a follow-up and looked like a new man! No more dark circles under his eyes, and he reported much better sleep, a boost in his mood and, crucially, he woke feeling refreshed and was able to enjoy time with his kids, helping with their bedtime before returning to his night shift. His headaches had resolved, and although he still struggled with the alternating day–night pattern, he knew what strategies worked for him to make it easier on his body and was happy to be able to keep working and supporting his family.

How to set a healthy sleep routine

Here are a few simple ways to reset your body's natural rhythm and begin to focus your attention on a routine that fosters a decent night's sleep:

- ✿ **Follow the light.** Light exposure is an important cue for your body and your circadian rhythm. Retinal ganglion cells in our eyes detect light and pass the information to the body's master clock – the suprachiasmatic nucleus – which tells the body to make more melatonin.[54] Follow the earth's natural cues, exposing yourself to light first thing in the morning and throughout the day, and then dim the lights in the evening as the sun goes down.

✸ **Create a sleep sanctuary.** I know the late-night look at your phone is so tempting – scrolling through news apps, social media, WhatsApp or emails rather than going to sleep. To be kinder to yourself and your body, make your bedroom a restful place. Why not use an old-fashioned alarm clock instead of your phone? You can charge your phone in the hallway or in another room to avoid the lure of that bright, colourful screen. Many people also benefit from blackout blinds, using eye masks and keeping their bedrooms at a cool temperature.

✸ **Normalise earlier mealtimes.** Metabolism and digestion play a role in your circadian rhythm. When you eat and what you eat can help you reset your body clock.[55] Allow a few hours between your last meal and going to bed, if you can. One study showed eating within three hours of going to bed increased chances of waking in the night and having disturbed sleep.[56] It is also important to limit caffeine after lunch.[57] If you like a hot drink in the evenings, herbal teas can be an excellent choice, particularly chamomile tea, which has a calming effect. Just be sure not to drink too much, as a full bladder can also disrupt sleep.

✸ **Sensible naps.** Many cultures around the world take a midday nap. Short naps can have many benefits, including reduced stress, improved creativity and increased alertness and performance.[58,59] The key to napping well seems to be short bursts of 5 to 15 minutes. If you sleep for longer than this, your body will enter a deeper sleep cycle and you may wake up feeling groggy. Early afternoon seems to be the optimal time for a nap.[60] If you struggle to get to sleep at night, or have a sleep disorder that means napping could prevent sleepiness at night, it might be best to avoid naps.[61]

✸ **Stick to a routine.** One of the most effective ways to sleep well is to follow the same routine every day, even at the weekends. Trying to catch up on late nights by having lie-ins just doesn't work on a physiological level. The body experiences it as a form of jet lag and is not able to 'catch up' as we would hope. Having a routine before you sleep, such as taking a bath, reading a book and then brushing your teeth, can also act as a signal to your body that it is time to sleep.

✸ **Move.** Exercise naturally makes the body more tired and will increase both quality of sleep and sleep duration. The best times to exercise are in the early morning or early to mid-afternoon because this will raise the body temperature slightly, allowing it to drop a few hours later and send a signal to the body that it is time to sleep.[62] It can be particularly beneficial to exercise outside, to let your body absorb sunlight.

Do any of these suggestions resonate with you?

Meditation for sleep

I'm a big fan of meditation. It is not included as a specific practice for much of the book, because unlike most of the simple habits I've suggested, it can feel like hard work to start with. The good news is, study evidence suggests that for people who had never meditated before, just 13 minutes of meditation a day (for eight weeks) can have significant benefits for reducing feelings of stress, as well as improving mood, attention and memory.[63] Other benefits discussed in the scientific literature include reductions in anxiety and physical pain perception, improved quality of life and, importantly for this chapter, improved sleep.[64,65] It may even be a strategy for lowering blood pressure and preventing dementia.[66,67]

Understandably, meditation can feel boring and frustrating, and many people decide it's not for them. I find it helps to think of meditation as anything that connects us to our deep inner self. This could be done through art, while running, in practising yoga or just by feeling grateful for the blessings in our life. It doesn't have to be sitting cross-legged like Buddha. But if you are curious about receiving some of the health benefits above, you might like to try a more formal meditation habit. Even five minutes a day, to start with, can be beneficial. You could try a mantra-based meditation, which is a repetition of a phrase or sound. This is a very common form of meditation used in various religions and in transcendental meditation. You could also try a mindfulness meditation, which involves being present to the physical sensations and thoughts of the current moment. There is good evidence to show mindfulness meditation is helpful for improving sleep.[68,69] This could be because meditation improves control of the autonomic nervous system (thereby reducing heart rate and blood pressure), and it may also increase serotonin (the 'happy' hormone), and melatonin (the sleep hormone, made from serotonin).[70,71]

Let's give it a go:

1. Find a quiet area. Sit or lie down, depending on what feels most comfortable. Lying down is preferable at bedtime.
2. Close your eyes and breathe slowly. Inhale and exhale deeply. Focus on your breathing. You can use the techniques from page 240.
3. If a thought pops up, notice it, let it go and refocus on your breathing.

That's it. As you try meditation for sleep, be patient with yourself. Start by meditating for 3 to 5 minutes before bed. Over time, you can slowly increase the time to 15 to 20 minutes. Remember to be kind to your wandering mind. It is the mind's job to wander. Don't aim to push all thoughts away. Just recognise them, and then refocus on your breath.

It is interesting to see what comes up during meditation. You may be more aware of physical sensations (things that touch your skin, smells and sounds), your emotions (*I can't stand that, I love this, I crave that, I wish this . . .*) and random thoughts (*If the tomato is a fruit, then ketchup must be jam . . .*). Enjoy what comes up. Remember that your thoughts are not you. They will come and they will go. The inner self (who notices the thoughts as they come and go) is what always remains.

If you want a phrase for your wandering mind to focus on, that you can slowly repeat, there are many to choose from. If you have a religion, a mantra-based prayer is useful. Examples include The Lord's Prayer for Christians, or the phrase 'maranatha' ('Come, Lord Jesus') from Aramaic; this phrase is often said in Catholic traditions with the help of a rosary (prayer beads). Reciting the shahada is the declaration of faith in Islam, and for practicing Muslims it is repeated five times a day, as the first pillar of faith. There is an ancient Hawaiian mantra practice known as Ho'oponopono, which simply means 'to make right or bring back to balance', and it is composed of four simple phrases. 'I'm sorry; please forgive me; I love you; thank you.' Simply repeating these phrases alongside slow breaths is a hugely powerful and healing meditation.

Here are three mantra ideas from Eastern religion and philosophy:

1. **'Oṃ'**
   This is the most sacred mantra in Hinduism and Tibetan Buddhism. In Sanskrit texts it has been described as the sound of creation, the original vibration of the universe. It is a soothing sound when spoken aloud, and has a wonderful vibration to it.

2. **'Oṃ maṇi padme hūṃ'**
   A powerful ancient Buddhist mantra, it translates as 'praise to the jewel in the lotus'. Each of the six syllables relates to the six goals of Buddhist living (and is represented on prayer flags all over the world).

3. **'Lokāḥ Samastāḥ Sukhino Bhavantu'**
   This is a Sanskrit peace mantra which means: 'May all beings everywhere be happy and free, and may the thoughts, words and actions of my own life contribute in some way to that happiness and freedom.'

It can be helpful to listen to guided meditations to get you started, or to perhaps listen to these mantras online if you feel drawn to one of them, as a way of recognising their sounds. You can just listen to them and let your body relax, or after a while you could repeat them back aloud or in your head.

Try some active relaxation

Qigong (pronounced 'chi gong') was developed in China thousands of years ago and is part of the Chinese self-healing tradition, or Yang Sheng. It involves using simple exercises to harness energy within the body, mind and spirit. You may have seen groups of people doing slow purposeful movements with their arms and legs in a park setting; this is likely to have been a qigong session in action. Qi is explained in many ways, but the easiest way to think of it is as 'energy', or perhaps 'life force'. In Chinese medicine it is considered to be the energy vibration that flows inside all living things. As we sit quietly, our bodies are actually busy keeping us alive; there are a huge host of metabolic processes going on: our hearts are beating, our intestines are digesting, our brain is keeping our lungs active so we can breathe in and out without needing to think at all. Each cell in our bodies is in constant motion, and it is this energy as well as the power of our breath, that combine to produce qi. Then, if we expand our understanding in this context, we will also be aware of the fact that all living things exhibit their own vibration pattern. In this way you can think of yourself as a wave but also as part of the ocean. Your qi is yours, but you share it with the planet too.

The 'gong' from 'Qi Gong' means 'work' or 'gather', and so 'Qigong' is like a moving meditation, and its proponents claim it can improve spiritual enlightenment, prevent illness and promote longevity. In studies, regular qigong has been shown to calm the stress response, and improve bone health, blood pressure and immune function.[72,73] For this reason, I thought it would be wonderful to include one of the most powerful qigong movements, called 'lifting the sky', for you to try, and see if you'd like to expand this and make it a regular practice of one to two minutes a day.

1. Stand shoulder-width apart and keep your eyes relaxed and half shut.
2. Bring your hands in front of your body with your palms facing the floor and bring your fingertips together until they are almost touching. Your arms should be slightly bent and your hands should be at the level of your hips.
3. Breathe out, engage your abdominal muscles and gaze at your hands.
4. As you breathe in deeply, press your hands down towards the floor.
5. Then, let them gradually come up into a half circle with your palms facing outwards, as though there was a large half ball between your chest and hands.
6. Keep following your hands with your gaze, with your arms slightly bent as your hands reach your forehead.
7. Then, push your hands upwards as though you are lifting the sky, and look up as you do so.
8. When you reach the top, you then breathe out as you move your arms apart and out to the sides, then gently bring them down in a big circle.
9. You can then let your arms and gaze rest, back in the position in which you started.
10. Repeat these simple moves in combination with the breath for a minute or so.

Your bedtime journal

This is one of my favourite sleep-improvement practices because it works so well. Much of insomnia is driven by an active mind. To keep us safe, our mind takes us on ruminations that our brain and body don't need. We worry about the events of the day, replaying conversations, revisiting fears and anxieties. We can fixate on a negative future that has no bearing on the present moment. This is where your special bedtime journal (what I call a 'bed book') will come in handy. When you worry about something, write it down here, or on a to-do list that you can come back to the next day, so that your mind feels it is dealt with. Writing down what plays on your mind at night will reassure your brain that your body can relax.

Making technology work with your health

We are living in a social experiment that is about a decade old, and one that is happening in real time. The experiment is on our collective consciousness. It is affecting the way our society functions and the way our brains develop, as a result of the dual influence of smartphones and social media apps.

There are huge advantages to connectivity online – it can forge the communities I have spoken about, and the availability of educational resources and information has never been richer. I have benefitted from social media platforms myself, and I am as tempted by the lure of checking my notifications as anyone.

But our exposure to 'fake news', the overstimulation of our brains and the collective comparisons we make to the highlight reels of other people's lives has also never been more pervasive. Having a smartphone is like having another person that we take with us wherever we go, a person that we use in every silent moment to fill our minds with other people's ideas and perspectives, or their idealised lives. In this way, we are also mined for information by tech companies and individuals, and we ourselves become the commodity, with companies harvesting our attention as well as our money. How do we get the best out of what modern tech has to offer without harming our sense of self or our ability to focus on the things that hold meaning for us?

There is no formula for this, and the sweet spot will vary depending on your comfort with tech, your reliance on it for work and your pre-existing social support structure. It will also depend on what you use social media for.

Many of us will scroll social media to distract ourselves, in an attempt to manage boredom. Research has actually found that we smile up to 30 per cent less when our phone is present.[74] I believe it is crucial for us to think about ways in which we can create distance from our phones to live happier, more fulfilled lives.[75] Creating these phone boundaries could also help our confidence, sense of control and feelings of alignment as well.

Tips for a healthy relationship with tech

- ❀ **Turn off notifications** (so you see messages and updates when you want to, not when your phone wants you to).
- ❀ **Try black-and-white screen settings** – this has been shown to reduce the lure of the smartphone and reduce the dopamine hit we get from checking our phones.
- ❀ **Delete apps** – this doesn't have to be forever. But think about whether you really need to check your email on the go. Is it an emergency or could it wait until you are at your desktop or laptop?
- ❀ **Put your phone away when focusing.** When something needs your full attention, your phone is a distraction that will set you back from your full potential. You will find your productivity is improved

dramatically if, in a moment of reflection or boredom, you have to stand up and go to a different room to check your phone.

❀ **Use a 'do not disturb' function.** Your phone will have a DND mode that will allow you to stop all notifications, calls and texts from reaching you when you don't want to be disturbed. This could be especially useful while driving or during mealtimes.

❀ **Charge your phone in a different room to the one you sleep in.** This reduces the temptation to scroll before bed (which we covered in the section on sleep) but also partially addresses porn use, which is a huge issue affecting intimacy and relationships for many people. One way to reduce the effect this could have on our lives is to make it that little bit harder to access.

Treating your phone like a person may be the first thing you do to help you create clearer boundaries about how much you want it to play a role in your life. Do any of these tech tips feel manageable? Which of them will you start with today?

My patient Mia was 14 when she came in to see me with anxiety and low mood. Her mum came with her, worried about her sudden withdrawal from family life, the late nights in her room, her reluctance to go to school and her rapid weight loss.

Mia struggled to make eye contact. After a while of asking a bit about her friendships and routines, it transpired that she was being bullied online by one of the girls in her Year 9 class. She had been shamed for some photos of herself that she had posted. She was feeling crippled by the embarrassment of it all and was having suicidal thoughts. She wanted to disappear. She would be up late into the night looking at the comments and trying to gain the approval of this girl and the others in her group.

After going to the school with these concerns and agreeing to several hours of phone-free time, Mia started to eat dinners with her mum and two younger brothers again. She and her mum planned a holiday together and by the next follow-up appointment, she told me she had decided to delete the social media app from her phone.

This allowed her the mental space to cope with some of the social isolation she was still experiencing at school, and to escape from it for a few hours. She also joined a local theatre group and made some social connections outside of school, which was a massive boost to her confidence as well.

For Mia, making different choices around tech allowed her to build resilience in other ways, and turned into the major shift she needed to start the journey to feeling better about herself again.

For insomnia – the scoop on CBT-i

Data shows that insomnia-focused cognitive behavioural therapy (CBT-i) works, and is considered the first line of treatment for insomnia.[76] It is also helpful to treat insomnia that is a part of dealing with another health condition that can impact sleep (anxiety, alcohol use disorders, bladder and prostate issues, chronic pain, etc.).[77] CBT-i focuses on exploring the connection between the way we think, the things we do and how we sleep. If you have been struggling with insomnia, I recommend you find a trained therapist to help guide you through a six-to-eight-session programme. Here, I will outline the principles of treatment and what to expect, so you can be familiar with useful thought patterns and habits when it comes to fostering a good night's sleep.

Firstly, its useful to examine our thoughts and feelings about sleep. A major problem with insomnia is the fear that it will affect you the next day. Negative, stressful thoughts about sleep worsen loss of sleep by causing frustration. This causes a stress response in the body that keeps us awake. The harder it is to fall asleep, the worse the anxiety becomes. Here are some examples of unhelpful thought patterns:

- ❋ 'I've woken up now, so I'll never get back to sleep.'
- ❋ 'I'm going to be a wreck tomorrow.'
- ❋ 'I must get eight hours of sleep or I won't function.'
- ❋ 'I cannot fall asleep without a sleeping pill.'
- ❋ 'My insomnia is going to cause health problems.'

Do any of these sound familiar? Another issue with these thought patterns is that they can lead to feelings of negativity about being in your bed. You may spend hours lying awake, trying to force sleep. Or you may have a habit of eating, watching TV, using your laptop or scrolling on your phone in bed. In CBT-i (and perhaps as a good rule of thumb for life in general!), your bed is only for sleep and sex. If you can't get to sleep, or if you're lying awake for more than ten minutes, the advice is to remain in a restful environment, but leave the bedroom. Then, when you are feeling tired, go back to bed. Your alarm should be set for the same time every morning, regardless of how much sleep you had, and it's best to avoid daytime naps.

Another important thing to be aware of is that insomnia actually makes you underestimate how much sleep you are getting. Time perception is altered when you are feeling stressed, and it's also likely that you will perceive light sleep (non-REM, also known as stage 2 sleep) as no sleep at all. So you are probably sleeping for longer than you think.

With this in mind, more helpful thoughts could be:

- ✿ 'I have spent time resting my body and mind, even when I have not been asleep.'
- ✿ 'I'm probably getting more sleep than I think.'
- ✿ 'Sleep needs vary from person to person.'
- ✿ 'I can do well even with just a few hours' sleep.'
- ✿ 'Insomnia is very common; it affects half the population at some point in their lives.'[78]

Another element of CBT-i treatment is actually sleep restriction. Why? Restricting sleep increases your 'sleep drive', making it easier for you to fall asleep and get into a healthy rhythm. It can obviously make you tired during the day, so if you have seizures or bipolar disorder (which can be worsened by sleep loss), this technique is not recommended. If your sleep diary shows you normally get four and a half hours of sleep, you'll be advised to go to bed for a maximum of five hours to start with. Once you spend most of the time that you're in bed actually asleep, you'll be able to increase the sleep window. A gentler version, 'sleep compression', is often used for older patients. It is a more gradual sleep-restriction technique.

Hopefully, these suggested thoughts and behaviours can help you, even if you are not in a position to seek the help of a CBT-i practitioner.

Your Get Well, Stay Well Plan

W e have covered a lot of ground in *Get Well, Stay Well*. I expect some of the science and advice we have covered will have resonated with you more than other parts. So how do you integrate it in a way that works for you?

The guide opposite is a reminder that shows you all of the daily actions mentioned in this book, and the six health habits they cultivate through daily practice. I'd like for you to choose one action from each of the columns to start bringing into your routine, with the aim of creating *your unique health framework*. Some people like to change everything at once, but most of us find that this is overwhelming, and we slip back into usual habits. Small and repeated actions daily are useful to maintain our new perspectives. It is better to do one thing a hundred times than twenty things once. A bit like muscle memory, the more you apply these ways of thinking, the more instinctive they become.

Remember, life is filled with challenges, many of them outside of our control. But I hope you now feel in a better place to face those challenges with the tools in this book. Remind yourself that you can do difficult things, and that it is normal and necessary to get the sense that some of these changes do not feel natural, or even comfortable, at first.

Some of the actions you want to try might be a one-off experience, for example, writing a meaning-maker letter (page 37). Others will be things that I want you to make a part of your routine.

If this feels like a daunting task, don't worry. I'll be holding your hand and guiding you step by step so you can make a plan that you are really happy with, and that you are excited to do every day. Once you have browsed all the practical tips you have read about in the table opposite, keep reading.

GLOVES daily actions guide

Gratitude	Love	Outside	Vegetables	Exercise	Sleep
Meaning-maker exercise page 37	Positive self-talk exercise page 71	Tips for a safe sun-loving lifestyle page 112	Good-mood food page 153	Breathing for stress – or a concentration boost page 241	Questions to help you determine the quality of your sleep page 261
Simple habits that encourage gratitude page 42	Positive role modelling page 72	Tips for breathing the biome page 117	Nutrients to focus on page 157	Relaxing breathing – for anxiety and insomnia page 242	Advice for shift workers page 262
Your journal prompts page 44	Love letter-writing exercise page 74	How to benefit from a blue mind page 119	Tips for no-oil cooking page 162	One-minute reset page 242	How to set a healthy sleep routine page 265
Tools for navigating loss and heartbreak page 46	Positive statements page 75	Cold-water therapy page 120	The plant points calculator page 164	Breathe and laugh page 243	Meditation for sleep page 268
Emotional tie-cutting exercise page 48	Forgiveness letter exercise page 89	Grounding exercise page 124	Tips for mindful eating page 169	Shake it off page 244	Try some active relaxation page 271
Tapping exercise page 53	Loving-kindness exercise page 90	Nature-based health tips page 130	Combat the bloat page 170	The four-minute anytime, anywhere workout page 246	Your bedtime journal page 272
A visualisation exercise page 58	Finding your values page 95	Tips for a healthy home page 133	What does 'food freedom' look like? page 183	Starting the day with a morning stretch page 250	Tips for a healthy relationship with tech page 274
Reframing exercise page 60	Prioritising your values exercise page 98	Tips for reducing plastic and chemical exposures at home page 137	Quick and easy recipes page 188	How to keep moving page 251	For insomnia – the scoop on CBT-i page 276

How to start

The next section is based on the conversations I have with my patients when I am working out how to get to the root cause of their concerns. Please set some time aside to answer these questions, and be open and honest with yourself. At the back of this book are blank journal pages for you to note down your thoughts. Feel free to truly make it your own.

How do you feel today?

What is on your mind, what are you struggling with and why have you turned to this book?

Your goals

What are you hoping to feel as a result of actioning the six health habits? This can be in relation to your body: vitality, fewer aches and pains, more energy, better skin or something else *and* in relation to general wellbeing, e.g. being more grateful, more present, more optimistic for the future, more in tune with the natural world, more at peace, more joyful . . .

Your current routine

What does a typical day look like for you? You can choose a weekday or a weekend day, or combine them both to give you more of an idea of what a typical week looks like for you.

Eating and drinking habits

Do you eat breakfast, lunch and dinner? What about snacks? Note down what you eat in the morning, afternoon, evening and night-time.

Exercise habits

Do you tend to go to a gym, attend classes, do weight training, or run, swim or walk? Do you have a sit-down or an active job? Are you a parent or carer? If you do no exercise, where could five minutes of movement fit into your current routine?

Outdoor habits

Think about how much natural light you get. Do you see the sun much? Think about how much greenery you see. Do you have access to views of greenery from your home? Houseplants? Screensavers with images of nature? Photos or pictures of the natural world?

Sleep habits

How well do you sleep? Think about how much time you spend resting, as well. How many hours do you spend in a quiet or low-lit space?

Your environment

Who do you live with? Do you have pets? Do you live with extended family, in a house share, or alone? Are you in a hostile or a loving environment? How many people do you speak to on an average day? Do you work in an office or from home? Is your space cluttered? Are you in control of the air quality? How much do you sit/stand? Who is in your support network? Who do you support? Is there anything you would like to change about your current routine?

Your timeline

Now it is time to think a little bit about how your past could be shaping what is happening today. Your medical and social history is unique to you. You may ask why we should look at things that happened years ago to help make a plan for now. It is important to be able to process and move through hard times rather than focusing on them. But sometimes this exercise really helps my patients to join the dots between certain events in their lives and their current patterns. They can begin to see where and when their physical or mental health challenges may have started. This can also help you to map out your own habits and where your lifestyle has changed over time.

Consider your timeline from when you were in the womb (if your parents can remember back that far) to now, as well as genetic factors that may run in your family. Then consider where you came in the family. Are you a blended family? The youngest of four? An only child? Are you adopted or fostered?

Think about social questions. Ask yourself: were you close to your mother growing up? What about your father? Did you have a good relationship with your siblings? What are these relationships like now? What about other relationship patterns in your life? In terms of your friends and significant partners – do you see any issues that come up for you, or any repeated patterns in terms of who you are drawn towards and the people you are surrounded by?

There may be a lot to consider here, and remember, this is not about 'fixing' anything, but about bringing awareness to areas of your life that could impact your wellbeing.

Now I want you to begin to think about some of your significant life events.

Recall:

- ❀ accidents
- ❀ operations
- ❀ periods of travel or moving home
- ❀ relationship or friendship break-ups and losses
- ❀ bereavements

- ❀ infections
- ❀ achievements
- ❀ birth of children
- ❀ illnesses of loved ones
- ❀ changes of career

I know this is a lot! What this process will do is help you build up a better picture of what has come before, which will guide you to know more about what you need to focus on moving forwards. Write your answers to this section down in your journal or at the back of this book – my patients tend to write more than they expected once they get started!

Your story

Divide your life up as best you can by decades as you write down your experiences. When it comes to pre-birth, birth and early years, it will be helpful to ask a parent or early caregiver what they recollect of this time if that is possible. It could also serve as a way to connect with them and allow them to reminisce about when you were young. What you write now about your current self will also be useful for you to look back on in future months and years.

In your journal or at the back of this book, write half a page about your experiences at each of the following ages:

- ❀ Prebirth, birth and early years
- ❀ Teen years

- ❋ 20–30 years old
- ❋ 30–40 years old
- ❋ 40–50 years old
- ❋ 50–60 years old
- ❋ 70 and beyond

Were there any important things that came up for you while thinking about your timeline? Have the goals you decided on at the beginning of this section remained the same after looking at your daily habits, your routines and your personal timeline? Write down your reflections in your journal or at the back of this book.

Now you have reviewed your goals, your current habits, your routines and your timeline, how did that feel? Hopefully you are noticing some patterns. This is going to help you decide what you want to prioritise in your life.

If you are unsure where to start, I'm going to explain some simple concepts in the coming pages that could help you feel clearer on where you want to begin:

- ❋ trajectory thinking
- ❋ identity
- ❋ habit stacking
- ❋ the power of three
- ❋ my *Get Well, Stay Well* suggestions.

Trajectory thinking

Some habits require repetition. This is because small changes don't seem to matter much. If you go to the gym every day for just a week, you are probably still unfit. If you study French for six hours, you can't speak the language fluently. The same principle applies for 'bad' habits too; eating one donut isn't going to impact your health. But if you eat one every day for a year, you'll start to notice the impact. If you have to work late and ignore your children for one or two nights, they'll forgive you. But if this is a lifetime of behaviours, they likely won't be close to you. As James Clear describes in his book *Atomic Habits*[1] (which I thoroughly recommend), tiny gains can accrue over time to define the quality of your life in 20 years. Time acts to magnify the margin between your desired outcomes and your daily habits. This means good habits make time your friend.

It is easy to get disheartened if you can't immediately see results, and progress is not linear. But think of some species of bamboo; it can barely be seen for the first five years of its growth, as it builds its root network underground. Then, within the space of just six weeks, it can grow 90 feet tall. Change takes years – until it happens all at once. Because of our habits. Aim to be proud of your habits, not your outcomes.

Identity

When your behaviours (habits) and your identity are aligned, you are no longer pursuing a habit, but rather, you are acting like the type of person you already believe yourself to be. So if you think in terms of goals ('When I reach 70kg, I'll be happy' or 'When I've learned the piano, I'll feel good') you are actually limiting your happiness to achieving the goal. The goal is not to run a marathon, but to be a runner. The goal is not to read a book, but to be a reader. The goal is not to learn the guitar, but to be a musician. When you identify as a type of person, you are more likely to follow through with a corresponding behaviour.[2] It works for negative identities too: 'I'm terrible with directions', 'I'm always late' or 'I hate the gym'.

When you notice a habit you want to change, don't tell yourself, 'It's just who I am.' Instead, decide who you want to be, and prove it to yourself with your habits. Habits are small wins in the game of life. The process of building habits is really the process of becoming yourself.

So ask yourself: 'Who is the type of person that I want to be?' For example, if your goal is to be a healthy person, ask yourself, 'What would a healthy person do? Would a healthy person walk or grab a cab?'

Habit stacking

Professor BJ Fogg talks about habit-stacking principles in his book *Tiny Habits*.[3] He tells us that one of the best ways to build a new habit is to identify a current habit you already do each day, then stack your new behaviour on top. This is known as 'habit stacking'. In his work, Fogg uses the term 'anchoring' to describe this approach, because your old habit acts as an 'anchor' that keeps the new one in place.[4] Examples of this include:

- ❀ jumping jacks while waiting for the kettle to boil
- ❀ press-ups in the bathroom after cleaning your teeth
- ❀ meditating for one minute with your morning coffee
- ❀ saying one thing you are grateful for as you sit down to eat dinner
- ❀ kissing your partner as you get into bed.

Can you think of *one thing* you can habit stack from *Get Well, Stay Well*?

The power of three

How do you integrate *Get Well, Stay Well* in a way that works for you? We have discussed trajectory thinking, identity and habit stacking. Now I want to share the power of three. It is a tool used to connect the human brain to ideas, and to make them easier to remember. Human brains respond to patterns, and three is the smallest number required to make a pattern, making it highly memorable.[5] The rule of three is commonly used in books and films. How many wishes was Aladdin given? How many Musketeers were there? How many bears did Goldilocks visit? Three.

The power of three is believed to be derived from oral story-telling traditions, but is now used in all sorts of contexts to create a natural beginning, middle and end. Things that come in threes are more persuasive. That includes speeches ('*Veni, vidi, vici*', meaning 'I came, I saw, I conquered' and attributed to Julius Caesar, and a 'government of the people, by the people, for the people' from Abraham Lincoln's Gettysburg Address); slogans ('Slip! Slop! Slap!', an Australian sun-safety campaign, and 'Stop, Look, Listen', for public road safety); and advertising ('A Mars a day helps you work, rest and play' and, of course, the cartoon mascots Snap, Crackle and Pop, from Rice Krispies cereal).

Now that I've pointed this out, you'll see the power of three everywhere. Focus on each of the six pillars of the GLOVES framework in turn for a moment. Using the power of three, I've simplified the six pillars of the GLOVES framework into three areas to keep things super simple – plants, peace and purpose. You can use these three categories as a guide to create your personalised three-point plan.

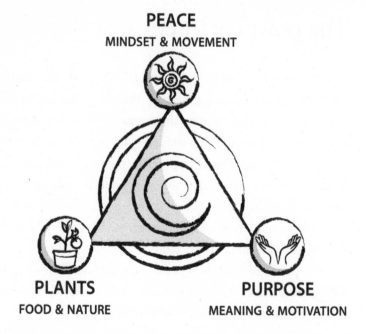

My *Get Well, Stay Well* suggestions

You might find it helpful to look at the suggestions I make on the following pages, which are based on the health struggles and health goals of my patients. They are combinations based on ideas my patients have found helpful over the years. If one really doesn't resonate with you, simply choose something else that does. You are in control.

Remember these are just pointers to get you started if you are unsure what you want to try. I have split them into two sections based on the book title. First up, suggestions for people who have specific health struggles in mind: the 'Get Well' section. This includes pointers for anxiety, asthma, back pain, high blood pressure, chronic pain, excess weight, depression, fatigue, gut problems, immune system issues, PCOS, type 2 diabetes and stress.

The second section is my suggestions for people with specific vitality goals in mind: the 'Stay Well' section. These suggestions are not exhaustive, but rather, they act as prompts to get you started. The vitality goals include better fitness, more focus, happiness, less loneliness, more connection, creativity and energy.

Also, it is important to note that if you have a medical condition, these suggestions for wellbeing never replace medical therapies. For example, I mention the power of effective breathing techniques. When you have asthma, clearly this would never replace the use of inhalers or oral therapies. I also mention depression, which is a clinical diagnosis requiring treatment that may include psychotherapy and medications; food or community-based suggestions would not replace treatments recommended by your doctor. This practical list is meant to be an adjunct to other ways in which you are also getting help – it is not an 'either/or' recommendation. You can use all the tools at your disposal to feel better.

Get Well ideas

Anxiety

Plants

Add in more herbs and spices for flavour in your cooking and for health benefits; ashwagandha could be a helpful choice to add to a smoothie, and reishi mushrooms are a lovely addition to your routine.

Limit caffeine after lunch. Does it make a difference to your sleep quality?

Go for a walk and pay attention to what you see, hear and smell.

Peace

Try talking therapy (via NHS online or in person, or privately) and try bedtime journalling for two weeks. See page 44.

Purpose

Do the tapping exercise (EFT) twice a week at moments where you need to shift your emotions, and notice your body feeling calmer too. See page 53.

Asthma

Plants

Get plenty of fruits and veggies for antioxidants. Omega-3s may reduce the production of immune cells associated with allergies (IgE production), which could improve lung function. Flaxseeds, chia seeds, hemp seeds and walnuts are great sources of omega-3s on a plant-rich diet, and algae oil is great for obtaining long-chain omega-3s.

Avoid synthetic fragrances and choose cleaning products carefully to avoid lung irritation.

Peace

Use a breathing exercise of your choice, daily (see page 240).

Switch from warm water to cold for the last 90 seconds of your morning shower.

Purpose

Consider joining a swimming group – outdoors or at a local pool. If you can't swim, could you take lessons? Or is there another leisure activity you could share with others and take part in each week?

Back pain

Plants

Prioritise olive oil, green tea and brightly coloured fruits and vegetables as part of an anti-inflammatory diet pattern that has been shown to reduce inflammation in cartilage, which helps to control back pain and stiffness. Green veg is great too; think of kale, spinach, and broccoli as A-listers when it comes to combatting inflammation.

Peace

Start the day with a morning stretch (see page 250) or practise the 'lifting the sky' qigong technique for three minutes twice a week (page 271).

Purpose

Actively curate friendships. Start to notice people that lift others or who seem to have values you admire. Make an effort to engage with them, or find ways you can contribute to their happiness without expectation of anything in return. You may find this lifts you too, and eases some of the tension you may be holding in your body.

High blood pressure

Plants

The nitrates in beetroot can help relax and widen blood vessels, which enables blood to flow through more easily, thus lowering blood pressure, so daily beetroot juice or fresh beetroot will be helpful. Try 2 tablespoons of milled flaxseed daily (it can be added to porridge, cereals, stews or salads), and two cups of hibiscus tea a day. See how your blood pressure is affected and consult with your doctor accordingly. Cut out salt wherever you can.

Peace

Try the forgiveness letter exercise (page 89) or meaning-maker journalling prompt (page 37).

Purpose

Check out the community gardens in your area – do you have time to share an allotment or grow food? You could analyse your work hours. Do you enjoy your work? What are you good at? What do people say they value about you? Spending time planning for a change of direction in your career, or planning for your future family, home or even retirement could really boost long-term happiness.

Chronic pain

Plants

Focus on daily portions of fresh or frozen berries on breakfast cereal, in porridge or as part of a smoothie. Another wonderful daily addition would be garlic, turmeric and rosemary, or perhaps a daily tea with black pepper, ginger and cinnamon, for their anti-inflammatory properties.

Peace

Try the 'lifting the sky' qigong technique for three minutes twice a week (page 271).

Plan a trip to visit the beach or a local forest.

Purpose

Do the values exercise on page 98 then practise your 'good guide' journalling prompt from page 73.

Excess weight

Plants

Foods such as kale, spinach and broccoli contain thylakoids, which have been shown in studies to curb hunger cravings.[11] Nigella seeds taken daily also seem to have similar effects – so if you enjoy them, these foods can easily be added to soups, stews or curries. Focus on staying hydrated and filling up on fibre-rich foods that will help keep you full for longer.

Eating an apple before lunch may improve digestion and keep you feeling sated. Remind yourself of the tips and promises in 'What does "food freedom" look like?' on page 183.

Peace

Positive self-talk challenge: notice your inner chat, write it down and turn it into what a good friend might say to you. You can use the journal pages at the back of the book to make notes.

Purpose

Start to notice people that lift others or who seem to have values you admire. Make an effort to engage with them, or find ways you can contribute to their happiness. The people we surround ourselves with can sometimes make or break our day-to-day happiness levels in surprising ways.

Depression

Plants

Simple swaps – Check out the 'Good-mood food' tips on page 153. Are there any foods or recipes you can eat each week that you weren't including before, to make sure you are hitting your nutrient goals?

Eat your food outdoors by taking a picnic to the local park or simply eating in your own garden or on your terrace.

Do you have the time for a pet? It is a way to encourage time outdoors and to bring more of the outdoors into your home.

Buy some fresh herbs in a pot at the supermarket and keep them on your windowsill. Water them and watch them grow.

Peace

Try the four-minute anytime, anywhere workout (page 246). Look up at the stars at night. You could even try to recognise different constellations.

Purpose

Role model mimicry. Write down the things your role model, if you have one, has done to inspire you (see page 73). Or if you know them, write the ways in which they talk to you and encourage you. Could you be that person to someone else? Could you remind yourself of their words when your negative self-talk starts to kick in?

Fatigue

Plants

Nuts and seeds are some of the best foods to beat fatigue; getting a variety of nuts and seeds in your diet can provide healthy nutrients and energy. Try almonds, Brazil nuts, cashews, hazelnuts, pecans, walnuts, sunflower seeds and pumpkin seeds. The perfect mid-afternoon snack!

Notice fractals outside and look at the sky each morning for five minutes.

Peace

Feeling tired and wired? Try Yoga Nidra. This is a form of guided meditation also known as 'yogic sleep'. It's usually practised lying down with a teacher guiding the session, but many guided Yoga Nidra meditations can be found online. Try a Yoga Nidra guided meditation every evening for seven days. Observe regular bedtimes and wake times daily. Limit naps if you struggle to get to sleep at night, or allow yourself a ten-minute nap if you find it helps your productivity.

Journal before bed.

Purpose

Once physical causes have been excluded, fatigue can sometimes come from feeling bored or looking for distractions in our lives. Try the values exercise on page 98 to reconnect with what gives you energy in your life. Reconnecting with loved ones could also help.

Sit at a table to eat with family or friends. This will encourage mindful eating, where you are in a relaxed state, fully present in the moment and able to take the time to properly digest your food, which may help with bloating and indigestion symptoms.

Write down one thing you are grateful for each day for one week.

Gut problems

Plants

Add some prebiotic foods to your routine to nourish your gut bugs, such as oats, underripe bananas, apples, flaxseeds, garlic, onions and leeks. If you bloat, head to page 170 for tips on how to help with that. Eat slowly and intentionally and enjoy every bite.

Get outside in nature – walk in a garden or around the block for five minutes before breakfast every day – and see how you feel.

Peace

Do the reframing exercise (page 60) every Sunday morning.

Consider a yoga practice, in person or online, or try the qigong exercise on page 271 as inspiration to join an online class.

Purpose

Sit at a table to eat with family or friends.

Try a routine at bedtime – what cues help you feel sleepy? Ideas could include taking a bath, reading a book or watching a calming and familiar show on TV with dim lights. These can all act as a signal to your body that it is time to sleep.

Immune system issues

Plants

Let's think about immune-boosting nutrients to include in your routine. Enjoy foods with high levels of vitamin C, zinc and protein – you could check out the comforting and delicious soup recipes in the Vegetables chapter on page 141 and eat a Brazil nut or two each day for selenium.

Peace

Could you spare 15 minutes a day to get some daily sunshine?

Try some of the cold-water therapy suggestions from page 120.

Purpose

Journalling. Do you want this to be free-flow writing, or specific to an emotion or event?

Think about whether the meaning-maker exercise (page 37) or the emotional tie-cutting exercise (page 48) could help you.

PCOS and type 2 diabetes

Plants

I've combined these two conditions as many of the drivers for both PCOS and type 2 diabetes are rooted in resistance to insulin. Focus on enjoying foods that do not drive insulin resistance (like veggies, fruits, wholegrains, legumes, nuts and seeds) and be sure to check your blood sugar levels regularly, as you may find that your insulin and medication requirements go down quickly. Great news, of course, but hypoglycaemia can be dangerous, so make sure your medications are reviewed regularly with these healthful dietary changes.

Peace

Try the four-minute anytime, anywhere workout (page 246) and incorporate movement with time outside wherever possible. Exercise is a great way to improve insulin sensitivity.

Follow the light – can you dim the lights after 8pm, for example, by using salt lamps or table lamps rather than overhead lights? I find rock salt lamps particularly calming. Avoiding the use of phones, iPads and laptops late into the evening will allow you to set your day–night rhythm. Avoiding late-night snacks will also improve your glucose metabolism and digestion. Setting your circadian rhythm and avoiding late-night snacks will also improve your glucose metabolism.

Purpose

Write down what value is most important to you today. Maintaining a healthy weight, movement and a good sleep routine are all helpful when living with insulin resistance. Reflecting on the value of health and what it means to you could be useful here. You can use the values exercise on page 98 to help with this. What could you do today to give you more health and vitality? Ask yourself this question for seven days in a row and see how this affects you.

Stress

Plants

Limit caffeine after lunch. Does it make a difference to your sleep quality? If you like a hot drink in the evenings, herbal teas can be an excellent choice, particularly chamomile tea, which has a calming effect.

Peace

Try the tapping exercise from page 53 daily.

Is there a way for you to let in more natural light to your home? Remember to open windows and curtains, and consider where light falls. Could your furniture or paint make a difference too?

Purpose

Clear out your wardrobe/declutter your home and give the items you don't wear or need to charity. Do the one-minute reset from page 242 for five days in a row. Do you notice a difference in your stress levels?

Stay Well ideas

Better fitness

Plants

Dried fruits (such as apricots, raisins and mango) give a concentrated source of carbohydrate, making them an energy-boosting snack. You'll also get a dose of fibre, potassium, phytonutrients, vitamins and minerals with every mouthful. Prioritise proteins with each meal; current research suggests that most athletes require between 1.2 to 2.0g of protein per kilogram of body weight, with endurance athletes on the lower end of the spectrum, and bodybuilders and strength athletes toward the upper end ($\geq$1.6g). Think about your 'BLT' foods (beans, lentils, tofu) and, of course, peas, nuts, seeds and protein shakes, if you want to.

Peace

Try a daily box breathing practice (page 241) to relieve stress and improve focus on your athletic goals.

Purpose

Visualisations and positive self-talk for events or personal athletic goals – think of the 'Who inspires you?' prompts from page 72.

More focus

Plants

Enjoy the smoothie from page 192 to nourish your brain, and include mushrooms in your routines. Medicinal mushrooms have important health benefits and studies show that lion's mane, reishi and chaga mushrooms are the three most effective medicinal mushrooms for brain health. They may help protect the brain and improve memory, mood, focus and concentration. I'm a big fan of lion's mane mushroom!

Get outside in nature each day, for at least five minutes, and regularly open your windows and doors for proper air circulation.

Peace

Create a sanctuary of your room. Could you get blackout blinds or a good-quality eye mask to help you sleep?

Purpose

Unplug. Do we really need to check emails and messages outside of the working day? Create an out-of-office email reply if you need to, so everyone knows you are not reachable.

Happiness

Plants

Try the Chocolate-date Bites recipe on page 197 to share with loved ones! Remember to boost your plant points each week – see the plant points calculator on page 164 to get started, and see if you can gamify the process to get a high plant score. Getting 30 plant points a week will make you the rock star of gut health!

Peace

Make time for laughter. Share a funny YouTube clip with a friend, watch a comedy film with your kids or even force yourself to laugh (as is done in laughing yoga) once this week. Do you notice a shift in your body?

Check out the list of suggested affirmations on page 76. Do

them daily for three weeks and notice any changes. If these don't resonate, try the 'good guide' journalling prompt on page 73.

Purpose

Pay someone a compliment every day for a week.

Do you have a loved one's birthday coming up? Generally, gifting people experiences (instead of material things) and making memories is more powerful than physical gifts.

Less loneliness

Plants

Can you make one of the recipes from this book to share at a coffee morning or suggest a dinner with friends? You can ask everyone to bring a dish of choice and see what yummy combinations your friends bring. Can you organise a social event if there is nothing local to you?

Peace

Join a local park run, or even parkrun UK (a series of free community events in the UK where you can walk, jog, run, volunteer or spectate). Do you know of a local walking group or social activity outside? If none of these work for you, could you text a friend to go for a walk or run with you?

Purpose

Seek to prioritise making a valued friend at work. Can you invite a trusted work colleague who you enjoy being around to come to your home for dinner? It is not always easy, but if you find someone you connect with, focusing on nurturing that connection can be done more consciously for a warm working environment.

More connection

Plants

Make a meal for friends or family, and if you fancy adding another creative element, make place settings or invent games for everyone to enjoy at a dinner party.

Peace

Promise yourself no phone time for the first 15 minutes of your day. Practise gratitude; reread the chapter starting on page 31.

Phone a friend once a week.

Purpose

Do you have time to volunteer locally? If you do, giving back to the local community is a lovely way to inspire others, boost your confidence or simply connect with someone new. What are you into? Sports? Star Wars conventions? Harry Potter? Find others who share those interests online or in real life to boost your wellbeing and sense of connection.

Creativity

Plants

It's time to experiment with some new recipes! Try any recipe from my book or the suggestions in the Resources section (page 317).

Encourage wildlife into your garden by using a bird box or bird bath.

Peace

Turn all notifications off for the apps on your phone.

Access your flow state – could dancing in the dark be something that gets you feeling free and creative?

Purpose

Keep a visual diary: take a photo of one thing that makes you smile every day. You could add it to a digital album on your smartphone, or a traditional album.

Try the visualisation exercise (see page 58).

Remember the magic of a role model. Can you reach out to someone you admire and arrange to thank them, or to meet up?

Energy

Plants

Bananas and chia seeds have both been shown to offer sustained energy for people with sporting goals – why not add them to a hearty bowl of oats and soy milk for an extra dose of slow-release energy and protein (from the soy milk) as part of your daily routine?

Peace

Try a routine at bedtime – what cues help you feel sleepy? Ideas could include taking a bath, reading a book or watching a calming and familiar show on TV with dim lights. These can all act as a signal to your body that it is time to sleep.

Purpose

Find your flow. Is there a job or a career that suits your natural talents and challenges you at the same time? Think about what might fit your identity (given your values from page 95), or that might benefit others. Remember happiness research suggests avoiding long commutes if possible. Can you bike or walk to work? If not, is it possible to get out for a walk in your working day?

The importance of awe and wonder

Professor of Psychology at UC Berkeley, Dacher Keltner has spent his career analysing the art of happiness. He credits the emotion of awe, and its pursuit, as being the key foundation for living a happy life.[6,7] Keltner charted emotions in a laboratory setting, and he has measured how they transform the way we think and act. This approach of looking from the inside out is especially apt when we consider that Keltner's work informed much of the Pixar animation *Inside Out*, the groundbreaking 2015 film which taught a generation of young people the importance of recognising our core emotions, and how they impact our actions. My favourite takeaway from the movie was an understanding of how central sadness is in learning how to cultivate empathy.

Peak experiences like 'flow', 'joy', 'bliss' or even 'enlightenment' are all similar, but what it really comes down to is a feeling of being in the presence of something vast that transcends your current understanding of the world. This could be something physical and external – like when you hear a singer's voice in an arena, look up into a clear night's sky, or stand next to a mighty oak tree in a forest. This could also be something emotional and internal – like the way you feel when you see a newborn baby's fingers and toes, or perhaps the feeling when you remember a taste or an aroma from childhood, or when you have a significant moment of connection with the story of another person.

Vastness could also be in relation to thoughts and culture – perhaps a sudden epiphany when things you didn't understand suddenly come together, or when you overwhelmingly feel a sense of belonging. The experience of 'vastness' is unique for each of us, and is also led by culture, but there are certain over-arching themes. We can feel awe externally or internally. External awe could be when we are in nature, looking at great trees, mountains, oceans and panoramic views. We can also feel awe at a rock concert, free-flowing dance experience, a wedding, a rally or even during a film. These are external sources of awe. But we can also feel awe internally, when we reconnect with ourselves through breath, laughter, movement, forgiveness and visualisation.

In *Get Well, Stay Well*, I focus heavily on gratitude, love and time outside, because awe can be generated from connecting with these feelings, and from paying attention to the beauty of the natural world around us.

How do you feel awe and wonder?

Your first *Get Well, Stay Well* plan

Now it's time to revisit the notes you made as you worked through the book. If you need to, gaining inspiration from my *Get Well, Stay Well* suggestions, you can now make your own plan of action. Grab your notebook or journal or use the journal pages at the back of this book and let's get started.

Using the ideas for plants, peace and purpose in this section, what is your first three-point *Get Well, Stay Well* plan? Write it down, then use the daily, three-week and six-week check-ins on the next few pages to reflect on your progress.

The one-minute daily check-in

I ask my patients to do this to help them stay focused on how they are feeling and how they want to feel. Write down (on a piece of paper, in a journal, at the back of this book or in the notes section on your phone) two things:

1. What could potentially get in the way today of you making healthy, happy choices?
2. What are you going to do to make sure you can stick with your goals as best you can?

Committing to asking these two questions each morning and writing down a brief one-sentence response to them is an effective way of keeping your goals in mind and sticking to them, whatever happens to come up. You'll have done a mini-mental rehearsal to help combat any foreseeable stumbling blocks and worked through them in advance.

Do this now.

The three-week check-in

Make a reminder to check in with yourself every three weeks. The process of making a note in your journal, diary, calendar or even on a sticky note on your desk or next to your bed will remind you to stay on track with your goals.

What are you noticing after your first three weeks? How are you feeling? What are you proud of that you tried doing/haven't tried before?

At around three weeks you may have found your motivation waning, your best intentions falling by the wayside. Don't worry – it happens to all of us. Rather than berate yourself, I would love for you to instead notice what went well this week, last week or the week before – what small wins can you celebrate?

Don't try to be perfect and don't worry if you fell back into old habits, just keep moving forward and feel good about every intentional choice. Remember, this is about adding value to your life, not going over and over the things you wish you'd done differently.

If you didn't manage to do all three things you promised yourself, notice the emotions this brings up in you. Do you feel something in your body, or have a critical voice in your head when you think about it? How does the self-criticism sound? What words or phrases come up for you and how will you respond to them?

Bring to mind someone you love or highly respect. If they did not quite achieve something they had set out to do, what would you say to them? How would you want them to respond to their setback? What could help them get back on track with it?

Write those thoughts in your journal.

Remind yourself of your values and code words (pages 95 and 100). What value is most important to you today? See page 98 if you need to remind yourself what you want to focus on at the moment.

What could you do *today* to serve what is most important to you?

The six-week check-in

After six weeks or so, are there any challenges coming up for you? There will no doubt be things you have noticed that did not go well over the last few weeks. There will also have been things that have already powerfully changed your day-to-day happiness in ways you had not expected.

Ask yourself: what have you enjoyed most so far? Are there any breakthroughs you have had, or recipes you know you'll come back to again and again?

Remember, it is natural and normal to experience setbacks. You deserve to feel good about yourself. Notice the habits that help you, e.g. getting to bed an hour earlier, five minutes of breathing, batch cooking – or whatever it is for you. Write a note in your journal about how you could add that habit in tomorrow, if it feels manageable.

Read this when you feel something is holding you back

The best-laid plans are often disrupted by the simplest of things. Change can be hard, especially with stress, time commitments, peer pressure, tiredness or any number of things getting in the way. If you have not been sharing *Get Well, Stay Well* with loved ones, your usual home routines – and changing them – will be an added challenge. Over the years many of my patients have said, 'I know what I need to do, I just can't seem to stick with it'.

Remember – it is normal, natural and necessary to veer off track, and to have hard days. Only when that happens can we begin to understand how best to gradually incorporate some of these new ideas into normality. Don't expect yourself to be able to do all of the things, all of the time. Just one thing – that's all you need to do to start with.

What one idea or routine from the three sections of plants, peace and purpose have you found easiest to stick with? Which one of those three things could easily become part of your normal routine today?

Your *Get Well, Stay Well* future

I'd love for you to start thinking about the future. What does life look like in the weeks to come after reading this book? Remember – you do not need to have followed it to the letter to have benefitted from it. A transition to a healthier lifestyle rarely happens overnight, but long-term changes can genuinely impact our health and happiness, as research with sets of twins has shown us.[8,9] We are born with around 20,000 genes, but the way they are expressed over time – and the microbiome that we develop as a result – has the power to alter our genetic destiny in myriad ways.

In fact, one study by Nobel Prize–winning scientist Elizabeth Blackburn indicated a healthy plant-based diet had the power to alter the expression of hundreds of genes that could improve the longevity of the cells in our bodies – even reversing the ageing process on a cellular level.[10] We also now know that the mind and body are not separate, and that our thoughts, our emotions and our actions are inextricably linked. Emotions play an important role in how we think and behave. The way we behave has the power to change our lives, the lives of those around us and, of course, our wider community and planet too. That's why your *Get Well, Stay Well* Plan is so important.

While, within our lives, we cannot turn back the hands of time, living to the fullest in the present is something I think we can all get behind. I would love for you to think about how you will reward yourself for keeping your *Get Well, Stay Well* lifestyle going six months from now. Which parts of the plan have you changed or added? How can you celebrate your new perspectives in life? What are you looking forward to?

What do you hope to be doing a year from now? Write down the future date in your journal or at the back of this book and tell yourself how you will feel.

Giving back

I have kept one last principle from *Get Well, Stay Well* until the end of the book. It is a secret that not many people know, and it is key to creating a more meaningful life. Earlier in the book we discussed ways in which we can experience more awe and wonder in our lives, and what that could look like for each of us. I saved one key area, the one in which we can feel the most awe, for last. According to psychologist Dacher Keltner's research, the thing that most commonly led his patients to feelings of awe and wonder was the inspiration provided by other people.

When we witness other people's strength, courage, acts of kindness or overcoming of adversity against all odds, that is when we feel the most awe and wonder. He describes this as a 'moral beauty', which is a goodness of intention or action, and is also the courage we show in the face of suffering. Perhaps you have a memory of feeling this way – maybe you have been in a situation of conflict and watched someone fight injustice bravely, or witnessed a loved one go through miscarriage, disability or disfig- urement, or face death with bravery or kindness? The amazing thing is that awe, wonder and happiness will often come from having been in a situation of pain or suffering. These are things we will all face. The way that we show up for these hardships will often be the very things that inspire the people around us in ways we least expect.

By making steps to improve your own health and happiness using the principles in this book, it is possible that you will allow others to experience a sense of awe and wonder by sharing your journey, your bravery and your vulnerabilities along the way. You will, in a real sense, be giving back to others and enriching their lives for the better as well as your own.

Throughout the book, we have talked a lot about practical

ways to instil your life with a sense of purpose. Happiness research tells us that we are social creatures, and that being around others, giving back to them and feeling accepted by them is a part of our sense of belonging.

Could you share these new habits and life changes with your friends, family or community so that they may also gain from you, and experience a more joyful life?

If your family or friends are resistant to changes, think about how you can accept this lovingly, and instead show them through your own happiness and health – and kindness towards them – how life-changing your insights have been.

Keep in mind – when the student is ready, the teacher arrives. You may be able to plant a seed of change in them, but the sun, the rain and the soil to let that seed grow may come from someone else, and that's okay.

Conclusion

Sometimes people are hard on themselves when they start out making changes. They can feel lost. Should we feel responsible for solving all the world's problems as well as our own? Absolutely not. Choosing to act in your own immediate reality is important. Feeling lost is actually an important part of that process, because it means you have begun to step away from the routines and patterns in your life that are not helping you. Feeling lost is a way of moving forwards.

Will things be perfect from now on? No! Life will not always go the way we want it to. Life is rarely a straight road, and we will face real hardship, sooner or later. The external world will never be perfect – and indeed that is not the goal here.

What this book will give you, I hope, is the freedom to notice your thoughts, your habits and where you have struggled up to this point. This book will give you the freedom to choose how to respond. The freedom to decide on routines that will help you, and make you feel good.

Your future is in your hands. Stay well, my friends.

Resources

Learning

The Plant Power Doctor by Dr Gemma Newman – your must-have, full-colour coffee-table book for general tips on plant-based eating, healthy and delicious recipes and specific science-backed information on skin conditions, hormone health, gut health, cancer, heart disease and immune health, as well as plant-based eating considerations for all ages.

The Proof is in the Plants by Simon Hill

Eating Plant-Based by Drs Shireen and Zahra Kassam

Vegan Savvy by Azmina Govindji, RD

How Not to Die by Michael Greger, MD

We Are the Weather: Saving the Planet Begins at Breakfast by Jonathan Safran Foer

Psychology and holistic health

Why Has Nobody Told Me This Before? by Dr Julie Smith

The Kindness Method by Shahroo Izadi

Feel Better in 5 and *The Stress Solution* by Dr Rangan Chatterjee

Why Woo-Woo Works by David R. Hamilton, PhD

The Blue Zones of Happiness by Dan Buettner
Ten Times Happier by Owen O'Kane
How Your Mind Can Heal Your Body by David R. Hamilton, PhD
Kitchen Table Wisdom by Rachel Naomi Remen, MD
I May Be Wrong by Björn Natthiko Lindeblad
Awe by Dacher Keltner
Yang Sheng by Katie Brindle
Lift Your Impact by Richard Newman
Atomic Habits by James Clear

Cookbooks

The Happy Pear: Vegan Cooking for Everyone by David and Stephen Flynn
The Seasonal Vegan by Katie White
Deliciously Ella Quick & Easy by Ella Mills
The 20-Minute Vegan by Calum Harris
Rachel Ama's Vegan Eats by Rachel Ama
Vegan Richa's Everyday Kitchen by Richa Hingle
The Plant-Based Diet Revolution by Dr Alan Desmond
Eat to Beat Illness by Dr Rupy Aujla

For specific dietary and health needs

The Fibre Fuelled Cookbook by Dr Will Bulsiewicz – a great resource for people experiencing potential food intolerances and gastro-intestinal symptoms.

The Plant-Based Power Plan by T. J. Waterfall – advice for athletes on a plant-based diet from an elite sports nutritionist.

Living PCOS Free by Dr Nitu Bajekal and Rohini Bajekal – a guide for people living with PCOS and insulin resistance.

Radiant by Hanna Sillitoe – focuses on plant-based healing for skin concerns and skin health.

The Plant-Based Dietitian's Guide to Fertility by Lisa Simon, RD

The Complete Guide to POI and Early Menopause by Drs Hannah Short and Mandy Leonhardt

The Health Fix by Dr Ayan Panja – a deep dive into a personalised health plan.

Deliciously Ella How to Go Plant-Based by Ella Mills – for great recipes and raising families on a plant-based diet.

Nourish by Reshma Shah, MD and Brenda Davis, RD – for parents raising their children on a plant-based diet.

Mastering Diabetes by Cyrus Khambatta, PhD and Robby Barbaro, MPH

The Alzheimer's Solution by Drs Ayesha and Dean Sherzai

For professionals

Plant-Based Nutrition in Clinical Practice edited by Lisa Simon, RD, Dr Zahra Kassam and Dr Shireen Kassam. A resource for dieticians, doctors and health professionals to understand the available data on the power of plants in nutrition. My hope is that books like these can help practitioners to feel confident in helping their patients and clients adopt a wholefoods, plant-based lifestyle if they choose to. I wrote the diabetes chapter in this book.

The Truth about Food by David L. Katz, MD, MPH

Rethinking Food and Agriculture edited by Amir Kassam and Laila Kassam

Proteinaholic by Garth Davis, MD and Howard Jacobson, PhD

A Prescription for Healthy Living: A Guide to Lifestyle Medicine edited by Dr Emma Short. I wrote the chapter on the benefits of fruits and vegetables for health.

'Plant-Based Nutrition: A Sustainable Diet for Optimal Health',
the University of Winchester's plant-based nutrition course. A
low-cost online course, and the only one that is focused on sustainable plant-based nutrition which is university accredited. I
wrote the diabetes section of this resource.

Websites

www.gemmanewman.com – links to further resources and *The
Wellness Edit* podcast.

www.theproof.com – a selection of evidence-based resources and a
podcast.

www.plantbasedhealthprofessionals.com – public and professional
health resources.

www.plantbaseddata.org/ – a library of resources on the benefits
of a plant-based lifestyle for the environment, health, prevention of zoonoses, economics and policy.

Acknowledgements

I have huge gratitude for the opportunity given to me by Laura Higginson and her team at Ebury, that I might share these messages with you. Laura believed in what I had to say, and gave tireless editing wisdom, for which I am truly so thankful. Thank you to copy editor Meredith Olson and Jessica Anderson for your hard work ensuring accuracy in referencing and clarity of word. Thank you to Rebecca Wheele, whose artistic talents have really made the book shine. I'd also like to thank Rowan Lawton and Georgina Rodgers, who both provided inspiration, advice and creative direction from the beginning. Thank you to Rohini Bajekal for inspiring recipes and conscientious review of early-days content.

A huge thank you goes to my mum, for providing recipes for my book that makes plant-powered foods delicious! You have always been so supportive of me, and let me know how proud you are. I am so grateful to you. Thank you to my cousin Freya Robinson for her noodles! Humble thanks also to my friends Ella Mills, David and Stephen Flynn, Dr Rupy Aujla and Katie White. They provided incredible recipes and inspiring stories that really lift this book's message and make it truly delicious.

For sharing their stories publicly, thank you so much to Tara Kemp and Adam Sud. You both shine with joy and purpose in the lives you have created, and the research and practical support you give to people is inspiring.

For content inspiration, I'd like to thank Shahroo Izadi, Katie Brindle, Dr Will Bulsiewicz, Dr Rangan Chatterjee, Dr Ayan Panja, Dan Buettner, Professor Dacher Keltner, Dr David R. Hamilton, Dr Shireen Kassam and Dr Venita Patel. I can attest to the fact you are all lovely people who I am honoured to know, or to have in my life. Thank you to Carmen, Rob and Carol for creating web links for the recipes. Thank you to Vicky Miles for making my life a lot easier, I am so grateful for your organisational skills! Thank you to all my friends, who ask me how the book is going (I can say it is finally finished) and who give me the honour of their time, support and company.

Thank you to my patients. You inspire me every day with your resilience, your humanity and your trust. I will never take you for granted, or the absolute honour I have in being your doctor.

Thank you to my husband, Richard. For 22 years you have been an intelligent guide and mentor, and I am only just beginning to understand the depths of your love for me. Thank you to our children, Max and Ted. I am so grateful you chose me to be your mum. I hope to do the best job I can. I learn from you both every day. Thank you to my dog Rosie: my shadow, my book-editing buddy and my little muse.

Lastly, thank you for the gift of life. In the words of Sharon Blackie, 'To live an enchanted life is to be challenged, to be awakened, to be gripped and shaken to the core by the extraordinary which lies at the heart of the ordinary. Above all, to live an enchanted life is to fall in love with the world all over again' (*The Enchanted Life*, 2018).

References

Introduction

1. Ellis, B., Ly, M., Steinberger, S., Chown, A., 'Chronic pain in England: Unseen, unequal and unfair.' Report produced by Public Health England and Versus Arthritis from data about population health collected by NHS Digital from the health survey for England in 2017.
2. Fulton, M. and Srinivasan, V. N., 'Obesity, Stigma and Discrimination', www.statpearls.com, 13 March 2023.
3. Stenning, A. and Bertilsdotter-Rosqvist, H., 'Neurodiversity studies: mapping out possibilities of a new critical paradigm.' *Disability & Society*, 36(9), (2021): 1532–37.
4. Truszczynski, N., Singh, A. A. and Hansen, N., 'The Discrimination Experiences and Coping Responses of Non-binary and Trans People.' *Journal of Homosexuality*, 69(4), (2022):741–55.
5. Watson, K. B., Carlson, S. A., Loustalot, F. et al. 'Chronic Conditions Among Adults Aged 18–34 Years – United States, 2019.' *Morbidity and Mortality Weekly Report*, 71(30), (2022): 964–70.
6. McManus, S., Meltzer, H., Brugha, T. et al., 'Adult psychiatric morbidity in England, 2007: Results of a household survey' (2007).
7. Green, H., McGinnity, A., Meltzer, H., Ford, T., Goodman, R., *Mental health of children and young people in Great Britain, 2004*. (Palgrave Macmillan, 2005).
8. McManus, S., Bebbington, P., Jenkins, R., Brugha, T. (eds.) 'Mental health and wellbeing in England: Adult Psychiatric Morbidity Survey 2014.'NHS Digital: Leeds (2016).
9. Medina-Perucha, L., Pistillo, A., Raventós, B. et al, 'Endometriosis prevalence and incidence trends in a large population-based study in Catalonia (Spain) from 2009 to 2018.'*Women's Health* (2022).
10. Agrawal, M., Christensen, H.S., Bøgsted, M., et al., 'The Rising Burden of Inflammatory Bowel Disease in Denmark Over Two Decades: A Nationwide Cohort Study.' *Gastroenterology*, 163(6), (2022) :1547–54.

11. American Cancer Society, 'Cancer Facts & Figures 2023', *CA: A Cancer Journal for Clinicians* (2023).
12. Miller, F. W., 'The increasing prevalence of autoimmunity and autoimmune diseases: an urgent call to action for improved understanding, diagnosis, treatment, and prevention.' *Current Opinion in Immunology*, 80, (2023).
13. Manzel, A., Muller, D. N., Hafler, D. A. et al., 'Role of "Western diet" in Inflammatory Autoimmune Diseases.' *Current Allergy and Asthma Reports*, 14(1), (2014): 404.
14. Oliva-Fanlo, B., March, S., Gadea-Ruiz, C. et al.,'Prospective Observational Study on the Prevalence and Diagnostic Value of General Practitioners' Gut Feelings for Cancer and Serious Diseases.' *Journal of General Internal Medicine*, 37(15), (2022): 3823–31.
15. Roll, R., *Finding Ultra* (Three Rivers Press, 2013).
16. Jurek, S., *Eat & Run* (Bloomsbury Paperbacks, 2013).
17. Brazier, B., *Thrive* (Da Capo, 2017)
18. Barnard, N. D., Goldman, D. M., Loomis, J. F. et al., 'Plant-Based Diets for Cardiovascular Safety and Performance in Endurance Sports.' *Nutrients*, 11(1), (2019): 130.
19. Trapp, D., Knez, W. and Sinclair, W., 'Could a vegetarian diet reduce exercise-induced oxidative stress? A review of the literature.' *Journal of Sports Science*, 28(12), (2010): 1261–8.
20. Sutliffe, J. T., Wilson, L. D., de Heer et al., 'C-reactive protein response to a vegan lifestyle intervention.' *Complementary Therapies in Medicine*, 23(1), (2015): 32–7.
21. Kim, H., Caulfield, L. E., Garcia-Larsen, V. et al., 'Plant-Based Diets Are Associated With a Lower Risk of Incident Cardiovascular Disease, Cardiovascular Disease Mortality, and All-Cause Mortality in a General Population of Middle-Aged Adults.' *Journal of the American Heart Association*, 8(16), (2019).
22. Kim, H., Caulfield, L. E. and Rebholz, C. M., 'Healthy Plant-Based Diets Are Associated with Lower Risk of All-Cause Mortality in US Adults.' *The Journal of Nutrition*, 148(4), (2–18): 624–31.
23. Turner-McGrievy, G. M., Wirth, M. D., Shivappa, N. et al., 'Randomization to plant-based dietary approaches leads to larger short-term improvements in Dietary Inflammatory Index scores and macronutrient intake compared with diets that contain meat.' *Nutrition Research*, 35(2), (2015): 97–106.
24. Najjar, R. S., Moore, C. E. and Montgomery, B. D., 'Consumption of a defined, plant-based diet reduces lipoprotein(a), inflammation, and other atherogenic lipoproteins and particles within 4 weeks.' *Clinical Cardiology*, 41(8), (2018): 1062–8.
25. Kim, M. K., Cho, S. W. and Park, Y. K., 'Long-term vegetarians have low oxidative stress, body fat, and cholesterol levels.' *Nutrition Research and Practice*, 6(2), (2012):155–61.
26. Alexander, S., Ostfeld, R. J., Allen, K. and Williams, K. A., 'A plant-based diet and hypertension.' *Journal of Geriatric Cardiology*, 14(5), (2017): 327–30.
27. Whelton, S. P., Hyre, A. D., Pedersen, B. et al., 'Effect of dietary fiber intake on blood pressure: a meta-analysis of randomized, controlled clinical trials.' *Journal of Hypertension*, 23(3), (2005): 475–81.
28. GBD 2017 Diet Collaborators, 'Health effects of dietary risks in 195 countries, 1990–2017: a systematic analysis for the Global Burden of Disease Study 2017.' *The Lancet*, 393(10184), (2019): 1958–72.

29. Liu, R. H., 'Health benefits of fruit and vegetables are from additive and synergistic combinations of phytochemicals,' *The American Journal of Clinical Nutrition*, 78(3), (2003): 517S–520S.

30. Ornish, D., Lin, J., Chan et al., 'Effect of comprehensive lifestyle changes on telomerase activity and telomere length in men with biopsy-proven low-risk prostate cancer: 5-year follow-up of a descriptive pilot study.' *The Lancet Oncology*, 14(11), (2013): 1112–20.

31. Shivappa, N., 'Diet and Chronic Diseases: Is There a Mediating Effect of Inflammation?.' *Nutrients*, 11(7), (2019).

32. Buettner, D. and Skemp, S., 'Blue Zones: Lessons from the World's Longest Lived.' *American Journal of Lifestyle Medicine*, 10(5), (2016): 318–21. Published 2016 Jul 7. doi:10.1177/1559827616637066

33. Kobayashi, J., Ohtake, K. and Uchida, H., 'NO-Rich Diet for Lifestyle-Related Diseases.' *Nutrients*, 7(6), (2015): 4911–37.

34. Cornu, M., Albert, V. and Hall, M. N., 'mTOR in aging, metabolism, and cancer.' *Current Opinion in Genetics & Development*, 23(1), (2013): 53–62.

35. Kitada, M., Ogura, Y., Monno, I. and Koya, D., 'The impact of dietary protein intake on longevity and metabolic health.' *eBioMedicine*, 43, (2019): 632–40.

36. Gentile, D., Boselli, D., O'Neill, G. et al., A., 'Cancer Pain Relief After Healing Touch and Massage.' *The Journal of Alternative Complementary Medicine*, 24(9–10), (2018): 968–73.

37. Lacorossi, L., Di Ridolfi, P., Bigiarini, L. et al., 'The impact of Reiki on side effects in patients with head-neck neoplasia undergoing radiotherapy: a pilot study.' *Professioni Infermieristiche*, 70(3), (2017): 214–21.

38. Mueller, G., Palli, C. and Schumacher, P., 'The effect of Therapeutic Touch on Back Pain in Adults on a Neurological Unit: An Experimental Pilot Study.' *Pain Management Nursing*, 20(1), (2019): 75–81.

39. Jahantiqh, F., Abdollahimohammad, A., Firouzkouhi, M. and Ebrahiminejad, V., 'Effects of Reiki Versus Physiotherapy on Relieving Lower Back Pain and Improving Activities Daily Living of Patients With Intervertebral Disc Hernia.' *Journal of Evidence-Based Integrative Medicine*, 23, (2018).

40. Vergo, M. T., Pinkson, B. M., Broglio, K. et al., 'Immediate Symptom Relief After a First Session of Massage Therapy or Reiki in Hospitalized Patients: A 5-Year Clinical Experience from a Rural Academic Medical Center.' *The Journal of Alternative and Complementary Medicine*, 24(8), (2018):801–8.

41. – Zins, S., Hooke, M. C. and Gross, C. R., 'Reiki for Pain During Hemodialysis: A Feasibility and Instrument Evaluation Study.' *Journal of Holistic Nursing*, 37(2), (2018): 148–62.

42. Doğan, M. D., 'The effect of reiki on pain: A meta-analysis.' *Complementary Therapies in Clinical Practice*, 31, (2018): 384–7. Epub 2018 Mar 10. Erratum in *Complementary Therapies in Clinical Practice*, epub 2021.

43. Midilli, T. S. and Eser, I., 'Effects of Reiki on Post-cesarean Delivery Pain, Anxiety, and Hemodynamic Parameters: A Randomized, Controlled Clinical Trial.' *Pain Management Nursing*, 16(3), (2015): 388–99.

44. Kwan, R. L.-C., Wong, W.-C., Yip, S.-L. et al., 'Pulsed electromagnetic field therapy promotes healing and microcirculation of chronic diabetic foot ulcers: a pilot study.' *Advances in Skin & Wound Care*, 28(5), (2015): 212–9.

45. Maté, G., *When the Body Says No* (Vermilion, 2019).

46. van der Kolk, B. A., *The Body Keeps the Score* (Viking, 2014).

47. Hamilton, D., *How Your Mind Can Heal Your Body* (Hay House Publishing, 2008).

48. Kaufman, S. B., *Transcend* (Tarcher Perigee, 2020).

49. Rippon, G., *The Gendered Brain* (The Bodley Head, 2019).

50. Lebreton L., Royer, S.-J., Peytavin, A. et al., 'Industrialised fishing nations largely contribute to floating plastic pollution in the North Pacific subtropical gyre.' *Scientific Reports*, 12, (2022): 12666.

51. Yoon, H., Lee, I., Kang, H. et al., 'Big data-based risk assessment of poultry farms during the 2020/2021 highly pathogenic avian influenza epidemic in Korea.' *PLoS One*, 17(6), (2022): e0269311.

52. Samreen, Ahmad, I., Malak, H. A. and Abulreesh, H. H., 'Environmental antimicrobial resistance and its drivers: a potential threat to public health.' *Journal of Global Antimicrobial Resistance*, 27, (2021): 101–11.

53. Moss, B., 'Water pollution by agriculture.' *Philosophical Transactions of the Royal Society Biological Sciences*, 363(1491), (2008): 659–66.

54. Ceballos, G., Ehrlich, P. R., Barnosky, A. D. et al., 'Accelerated modern human-induced species losses: Entering the sixth mass extinction.' *Science Advances*, 1(5), (2015): e1400253.

55. Poore, J. and Nemecek, T., 'Reducing food's environmental impacts through producers and consumers.' *Science*, 360(6392), (2018): 987–92. Erratum in *Science*, 363(6429), (2019).

56. The EAT-*Lancet* Commission on Food, Planet, Health, 'EAT-*Lancet* Commission', https://eatforum.org/eat-lancet-commission/eat-lancet-commission-summary-report/ (2019).

Gratitude

1. Sansone, R. A. and Sansone, L. A., 'Gratitude and well being: the benefits of appreciation.' *Psychiatry*, 7(11), (2010): 18–22.

2. Karns, C. M., Moore III, W. E. and Mayr, U., 'The Cultivation of Pure Altruism via Gratitude: A Functional MRI Study of Change with Gratitude Practice.' *Frontiers in Human Neuroscience*, 11, (2017).

3. Zahn, R., Moll, J., Paiva, M. et al., 'The Neural Basis of Human Social Values: Evidence from Functional MRI.' *Cerebral Cortex*, 19(2), (2009): 276–83.

4. Wood, A. M., Joseph, S., Lloyd, J. and Atkins, S., 'Gratitude influences sleep through the mechanism of pre-sleep cognitions.' *Journal of Psychosomatic Research*, 66(1), (2009): 43–8.

5. Alkozei, A., Smith, R., Kotzin, M. D. et al., 'The Association Between Trait Gratitude and Self-Reported Sleep Quality Is Mediated by Depressive Mood State.' *Behavioral Sleep Medicine*, 17(1), (2019): 41–8.

6. Ong, A. D., Zautra, A. J. and Reid, M. C., 'Psychological resilience predicts decreases in pain catastrophizing through positive emotions.' *Psychology and Aging*, 25(3), (2010): 516–23.

7. Pulvers, K. and Hood, A., 'The Role of Positive Traits and Pain Catastrophizing in Pain Perception.' *Current Pain and Headache Reports*, 17(330), (2013).

8. Mills, P. J., Wilson, K., Punga, M. A. et al., 'The Role of Gratitude in Well-being in Asymptomatic Heart Failure Patients.' *Integrative Medicine*, 14(1), (2015): 51.

9. Wong, Y. J., Owen, J., Gabana, N., et al., 'Does gratitude writing improve the mental health of psychotherapy clients? Evidence from a randomized controlled trial.' *Psychotherapy Research*, 28(2), (2016): 1–11.

10. Fritz, M. M., Armenta, C. N., Walsh, L. C. and Lyubomirsky, S., 'Gratitude facilitates healthy eating behavior in adolescents and young adults.' *Journal of Experimental Social Psychology*, 81, (2018): 4–14.

11. Tala, Á., 'Gracias por todo: Una revisión sobre la gratitud desde la neurobiología a la clínica [Thanks for everything: a review on gratitude from neurobiology to clinic].' *Revista Médica de Chile*, 147(6), (2019): 755–61.

12. O'Connell, B. H., O'Shea, D. and Gallagher, S., 'Feeling Thanks and Saying Thanks: A Randomized Controlled Trial Examining If and How Socially Oriented Gratitude Journals Work.' *Journal of Clinical Psychology*, 73(10), (2017): 1280–1300.

13. Martínez, M. P., Sánchez, A. I., Miró, E. et al., 'Relationships between physical symptoms, emotional distress, and pain appraisal in fibromyalgia: the moderator effect of alexithymia.' *The Journal of Psychology*, 149(2), (2015): 115–40.

14. Bekhuis, E., Gol, J., Burton, C. and Rosmalen, J., 'Patients' descriptions of the relation between physical symptoms and negative emotions: a qualitative analysis of primary care consultations.' *British Journal of General Practice*, 70(691), (2020): e78–e85.

15. Fredrickson, B. L. and Branigan, C., 'Positive emotions broaden the scope of attention and thought-action repertoires.' *Cognition and Emotion*, 19(3), (2005): 313–32.

16. Wadlinger, H. A. and Isaacowitz, D. M., 'Positive mood broadens visual attention to positive stimuli.' *Motivation and Emotion*, 30(1), (2006): 87–99.

17. https://worlddatabaseofhappiness.eur.nl/

18. Buettner, D. andSkemp, S., 'Blue Zones: Lessons from the World's Longest Lived.' *American Journal of Lifestyle Medicine*, 10(5), (2016): 318–21.

19. Veenhoven, R., 'Distributional findings on happiness in nations, sorted by nation, measure type and year.' *World Database of Happiness*, Erasmus University Rotterdam, The Netherlands. https://worlddatabaseofhappiness.eur.nl/

20. Hoffman, T., Bar-Shalita, T., Granovsky, Y. et al., 'Indifference or hypersensitivity? Solving the riddle of the pain profile in individuals with autism.' *Pain* 164(4), (2023): 791–803.

21. Clauw, D. J., Arnold, L. M. and McCarberg, B. H.; FibroCollaborative, 'The science of fibromyalgia.' *Mayo Clinic Proceedings*, 86(9), (2011): 907–11.

22. Ruggieri, V., 'Autismo, depresión y riesgo de suicidio [Autism, depression and risk of suicide].' *Medicina (B Aires)*, 80 (Suppl 2), (2020): 12–16.

23. Yepez, D., Grandes, X. A., Manjunatha, R. T. et al., 'Fibromyalgia and Depression: A Literature Review of Their Shared Aspects.' *Cureus*, 14(5), (2022): e24909.

24. Chellappa, S. L. and Aeschbach, D., 'Sleep and anxiety: From mechanisms to interventions.' *Sleep Medicine Reviews*, 61, (2022): 101583.

25. Van Laarhoven, A. I. M., Walker, A. L., Wilder-Smith, O. H. et al., 'Role of induced negative and positive emotions in sensitivity to itch and pain in women.' *British Journal of Dermatology*, 167(2), (2012): 262–69.

26. Emmons, R. A. and McCullough, M. E., 'Counting Blessings Versus Burdens: An Experimental Investigation of Gratitude and Subjective Well-being in Daily Life.' *Journal of Personality and Social Psychology*, 84(2), (2003): 377–89.

27. Leknes, S. and Tracey, I., 'A common neurobiology for pain and pleasure.' *Nature Reviews Neuroscience*, 9(4), (2008): 314–20.

28. Norris, C. J., 'The negativity bias, revisited: Evidence from neuroscience measures and an individual differences approach.' *Social Neuroscience*, 16(1), (2021): 68–82.

29. Fredrickson, B. L. and Levenson, R. W., 'Positive Emotions Speed Recovery from the Cardiovascular Sequelae of Negative Emotions.' *Cognition and Emotion*, 12(2), (1998): 191–220.

30. Ostir, G. V., Markides, K. S., Black, S. A. and Goodwin, J. S., 'Emotional well-being predicts subsequent functional independence and survival.' *Journal of the American Geriatrics Society*, 48(5), (2000): 473–8.

31. van der Kolk, B. A., Stone, L., West, J., Rhodes, A. et al., 'Yoga as an adjunctive treatment for posttraumatic stress disorder: a randomized controlled trial.' *The Journal of Clinical Psychiatry*, 75(6), (2014): e559–65.

32. Valiente-Gómez, A, Moreno-Alcázar, A., Treen, D., et al., V. 'EMDR beyond PTSD: A Systematic Literature Review.' *Frontiers in Psychology*, 8, (2017).

33. Bach, D., Groesbeck, G., Stapleton, P. et al., 'Clinical EFT (Emotional Freedom Techniques) Improves Multiple Physiological Markers of Health.' *Journal of Evidence-Based Integrative Medicine*, (2019).

34. Yao, W. X., Ranganathan, V. K., Allexandre, D. et al., 'Kinesthetic imagery training of forceful muscle contractions increases brain signal and muscle strength.' *Frontiers in Human Neuroscience*, 7, (2013): 561.

35. Horikawa, T., Cowen, A. S., Keltner, D. and Kamitani, Y., 'The Neural Representation of Visually Evoked Emotion Is High-Dimensional, Categorical, and Distributed across Transmodal Brain Regions.' *iScience*, 23(5), (2020): 101060.

36. The Imagination and Health. *Edinb Med J*. 1888;34(5):486.

37. Slimani, M., Tod, D., Chaabene, H. et al., 'Effects of Mental Imagery on Muscular Strength in Healthy and Patient Participants: A Systematic Review.' *Journal of Sports Science & Medicine*, 15(3), (2016): 434–50.

38. Wright, L. M., 'Brain science and illness beliefs: an unexpected explanation of the healing power of therapeutic conversations and the family interventions that matter.' *Journal of Family Nursing*, 21(2), (2015): 186–205.

39. Mobley, D., Baum, N. H., Beattie, A. and Nemeroff, C., 'When Imagination Becomes a Disease: Dealing with Hypochondriacal Patients in Clinical Practice.' *Ochsner Journal*, 19(2), (2019): 70–3.

40. Finniss, D. G., Kaptchuk, T. J., Miller, F. and Benedetti, F., 'Biological, clinical, and ethical advances of placebo effects.' *The Lancet*, 375(9715), (2010): 686–95.

41. Chatterjee, R., *Feel Better In 5* (Penguin Life, 2019).

Love

1. Research Institute of Molecular Pathology, 'The biology of emotions.' *ScienceDaily*, 17 September 2012, https://www.sciencedaily.com/releases/2012/09/120917111056.htm.

2. National Research Council (US) Panel to Review the Status of Basic Research on School-Age Children; Collins, W. A., (ed.), 'Chapter 3: Cognitive Development in School Age Children: Conclusions and New Directions' in *Development During Middle Childhood: The Years from Six to Twelve* (National Academies Press (US), 1984).

3. Johnson, R. A., *Owning Your Own Shadow* (Thorsons, 1992).

4. Millard, L. A., Wan, M. W., Smith, D. M. and Wittkowski, A., 'The effectiveness of compassion focused therapy with clinical populations: A systematic review and meta-analysis.' *Journal of Affective Disorders*, 326, (2023): 168–92.

5. Hill, N., *Think and Grow Rich* (Capstone, 2009).

6. Kross, E., Bruehlman-Senecal, E., Park, J. et al., 'Self-talk as a regulatory mechanism: how you do it matters.' *Journal of Personality and Social Psychology*, 106(2), (2014): 304–24.

7. Stroud, M. W., Thorn, B. E., Jensen, M. P. and Boothby, J. L., 'The relation between pain beliefs, negative thoughts, and psychosocial functioning in chronic pain patients.' *Pain*, 84(2–3), (2000): 347–52.

8. Finan, P. H. and Garland, E. L., 'The role of positive affect in pain and its treatment.' *The Clinical Journal of Pain*, 31(2), (2015): 177–87.

9. Tangney, J. P., Stuewig, J. and Martinez, A. G., 'Two faces of shame: the roles of shame and guilt in predicting recidivism.' *Psychological Science*, 25(3), (2014): 799–805.

10. Turner, J. C., Oakes, P. J., Haslam, S. A. and McGarty, C., 'Self and Collective: Cognition and Social Context.' *Personality and Social Psychology Bulletin*, 20(5), (1994): 454–63.

11. Department for Culture, Media and Sport, *Tackling loneliness evidence review: executive summary*, 17 March 2023, https://www.gov.uk/government/publications/tackling-loneliness-evidence-review/tackling-loneliness-evidence-review-summary-report.

12. Holt-Lunstad, J., Smith, T. B., Baker, M. et al., 'Loneliness and social isolation as risk factors for mortality: a meta-analytic review.' *Perspectives on Psychological Science*, 10(2), (2015): 227–37.

13. Long, R. M., Terracciano, A., Sutin, A. R. et al., 'Loneliness, Social Isolation, and Living Alone Associations with Mortality Risk in Individuals Living with Cardiovascular Disease: A Systematic Review, Meta-Analysis, and Meta-Regression.' *Psychosomatic Medicine*, 85(1), (2023): 8–17.

14. Freedman, A. and Nicolle, J., 'Social isolation and loneliness: the new geriatric giants: Approach for primary care.' *Canadian Family Physician*, 66(3), (2020): 176–82.

15. Perissinotto, C. M., Stijacic Cenzer, I. and Covinsky, K. E., 'Loneliness in Older Persons: A predictor of functional decline and death.' *Archives of Internal Medicine*, 172(14), (2012): 1078–83.

16. Kim, M. J., Loucks, R. A., Palmer, A. L. et al., 'The structural and functional connectivity of the amygdala: From normal emotion to pathological anxiety.' *Behavioural Brain Research*, 223(2), (2011): 403–10.

17. Stein, M., Keller, S. E. and Schleifer, S. J., 'Immune system. Relationship to anxiety disorders.' *Psychiatric Clinics of North America*, 11(2), (1998): 349–60.

18. Rokach, A., Sha'ked, A. and Ben-Artzi, E., 'Loneliness in Intimate Relationships Scale (LIRS): Development and Validation.' *International Journal of Environmental Research and Public Health*, 19(19), (2022): 12970.

19. Winston, R. and Chicot, R., 'The importance of early bonding on the long-term mental health and resilience of children.' *London Journal of Primary Care*, 8(1), (2016): 12–14.

20. Buettner, D., *The Blue Zones of Happiness* (National Geographic, 2017).

21. Spencer-Hwang, R., Torres, X., Valladares, J. et al., 'Adverse Childhood Experiences among a Community of Resilient Centenarians and Seniors: Implications for a Chronic Disease Prevention Framework.' *The Permanente Journal*, 22(2), (2018).

22. Yeung, J. W. K., Zhang, Z. and Kim, T.Y., 'Volunteering and health benefits in general adults: cumulative effects and forms.' *BMC Public Health*, 18, (2018): 8.
23. Provine, R. R., *Laughter: A Scientific Investigation* (Viking, 2000).
24. BMJ Specialty Journals. 'Comedy Films Boost Blood Flow to The Heart.' *ScienceDaily*, 18 January 2006, https://www.sciencedaily.com/releases/2006/01/060118095009.htm.
25. Lacoboni, M., 'Imitation, empathy, and mirror neurons.' *Annual Review of Psychology*, 60, (2009): 653–70.
26. Conway, C. A., Jones, B. C., DeBruine, L. M. and Little, A. C., 'Evidence for adaptive design in human gaze preference.' *Proceedings of the Royal Society Biological Sciences*, (1630), (2008): 63–9.
27. McCullough, M. E., Pargament, K. I. and Thoresen, C. E. (eds.), *Forgiveness: Theory, Research, and Practice* (Guilford Press, 2001), pp. 254–80.
28. Worthington Jr., E. L. and Scherer, M., 'Forgiveness is an emotion-focused coping strategy that can reduce health risks and promote health resilience: Theory, review, and hypotheses.' *Psychology and Health*, 19(3), (2004): 385–405.
29. WorthingtonJr, E. L., van Oyen Witvliet, C., Lerner, A. J. and Scherer, M., 'Forgiveness in health research and medical practice.' *Explore*,1(3), (2005): 169–76.
30. Lee, Y.-R. and Enright, R. D., 'A Forgiveness Intervention for Women With Fibromyalgia Who Were Abused in Childhood: A Pilot Study.' *Spirituality in Clinical Practice*, 1(3), (2014): 203–17.
31. Wilson, T., Milosevic, A., Carroll, M. et al., 'Physical Health Status in Relation to Self-Forgiveness and Other-Forgiveness in Healthy College Students.' *Journal of Health Psychology*, 13(6), (2008): 798–803.
32. Remen, R. N., *Kitchen Table Wisdom: Stories That Heal* (Riverhead Books, 1996).
33. Boreham I.D., Schutte N.S., 'The relationship between purpose in life and depression and anxiety: A meta-analysis.' *J Clin Psychol*. 2023 August 12. doi: 10.1002/jclp.23576. Epub ahead of print. PMID: 37572371.
34. Li, F., Chen, J., Yu, L. et al., 'The Role of Stress Management in the Relationship between Purpose in Life and Self-Rated Health in Teachers: A Mediation Analysis.' *International Journal of Environmental Research and Public Health*, 13(7), (2016): 719.
35. Hill, P. L., Edmonds, G. W., Peterson, M. et al., 'Purpose in Life in Emerging Adulthood: Development and Validation of a New Brief Measure.' *The Journal of Positive Psychology*, 11(3), (2016): 237–45.
36. Musich, S., Wang, S. S., Kraemer, S. et al., 'Purpose in Life and Positive Health Outcomes Among Older Adults.' *Population Health Management*, 21(2), (2018): 139–47.
37. Zilioli, S., Slatcher, R. B., Ong, A. D. and Gruenewald, T. L., 'Purpose in Life Predicts Allostatic Load Ten Years Later.' *Journal of Psychosomatic Research*, 79(5), (2015): 451–57.
38. Boyle, P. A., Buchman, A. S., Wilson, R. S. et al., 'Effect of purpose in life on the relation between Alzheimer disease pathologic changes on cognitive function in advanced age.' *Archives of General Psychiatry*, 69(5), (2012): 499–504.
39. Frisch, J. U., Häusser, J. A. and Mojzisch, A., 'The Trier Social Stress Test as a paradigm to study how people respond to threat in social interactions.' *Frontiers in Psychology*, 6, (2015): 14.
40. Smith, J., *Why Has Nobody Told Me This Before?* (Michael Joseph, 2022).
41. Newman, R., *Lift Your Impact* (McGraw Hill, 2023).

Outside

1. Weller, R. B., 'Sunlight Has Cardiovascular Benefits Independently of Vitamin D.' *Blood Purification*, 41(1–3), (2016): 130–34.
2. Wright, F. and Weller, R. B., 'Risks and benefits of UV radiation in older people: More of a friend than a foe?' *Maturitas*, 81(4), (2015): 425–31.
3. Holick, M. F., 'High prevalence of vitamin D inadequacy and implications for health.' *Mayo Clinic Proceedings*, 81(3), (2006): 353–73.
4. Holick, M. F., 'Sunlight and vitamin D for bone health and prevention of auto-immune diseases, cancers, and cardiovascular disease.' *The American Journal of Clinical Nutrition*, 80(6), (2004): 1678S–88S.
5. Llewellyn, D. J., Langa, K. M. and Lang, I. A., 'Serum 25-Hydroxyvitamin D Concentration and Cognitive Impairment.' *Journal of Geriatric Psychiatry and Neurology*, 22(3), (2008): 188–95.
6. Sansone, R. A. and Sansone, L. A., 'Sunshine, Serotonin, and Skin: A Partial Explanation for Seasonal Patterns in Psychopathology?' *Innovations in Clinical Neuroscience*, 10(7–8), (2013): 20–4.
7. Spindelegger, C., Stein, P., Wadsak, W. et al., 'Light-dependent alteration of serotonin-1A receptor binding in cortical and subcortical limbic regions in the human brain.' *The World Journal of Biological Psychiatry*, 13(6), (2012): 413–22.
8. Angerer, P., Schmook, R., Elfantel, I. and Li, J., 'Night Work and the Risk of Depression.' *Deutsches Ärzteblatt International*, 114(24), (2017): 404–11.
9. Lee, A., Myung, S.K., Cho, J. J. et al., 'Night Shift Work and Risk of Depression: Meta-analysis of Observational Studies.' *Journal of Korean Medical Science*, 32(7), (2017): 1091–6.
10. Bedrosian, T. A. and Nelson, R. J., 'Timing of light exposure affects mood and brain circuits.' *Translational Psychiatry*, 7(1), (2017): e1017.
11. Wilson, N., 'Depression and its relation to light deprivation.' *The Psychoanalytic Review*, 89(4), (2005): 557–67.
12. Wehr, T. A., Sack, D., Rosenthal, N. et al., 'Circadian rhythm disturbances in manic-depressive illness.' *Federation Proceedings*, 42(11), (1983): 2809–14.
13. Henriksen, T. E., Skrede, S., Fasmer, O. B. et al., 'Blue-blocking glasses as additive treatment for mania: a randomized placebo-controlled trial.' *Bipolar Disorders*, 18(3), (2016): 221–32.
14. Murray, K., Godbole, S., Natarajan, L. et al., 'The relations between sleep, time of physical activity, and time outdoors among adult women.' *PLoS One*, 12(9), (2017): e0182013.
15. Hardeland, R., 'Chronobiology of Melatonin beyond the Feedback to the Suprachiasmatic Nucleus – Consequences to Melatonin Dysfunction.' *International Journal of Molecular Sciences*, 14(3), (2013): 5817–41.
16. Rodella, L. F., Favero, G., Foglio, E. et al., 'Vascular endothelial cells and dysfunctions: role of melatonin.' *Frontiers in Bioscience-Elite*, 5(1), (2013): 119–29.
17. Srinivasan, V., Maestroni, G. J. M., Cardinali, D. P. et al., 'Melatonin, immune function and aging.' *Immunity & Ageing*, 2, (2005): 17.
18. Piccinetti, C. C., Migliarini, B., Olivotto, I. et al., 'Melatonin and Peripheral Circuitries: Insights on Appetite and Metabolism in *Danio Rerio*.' *Zebrafish*, 10(3), (2013): 275–82.
19. Blume, C., Garbazza, C. and Spitschan, M., 'Effects of light on human circadian rhythms, sleep and mood.' *Somnologie*, 23(3), (2019): 147–56.

20. Shechter, A., Kim, E.W., St-Onge, M.-P. and Westwood, A. J., 'Blocking noctur-nal blue light for insomnia: A randomized controlled trial.' *Journal of Psychiatric Research*, 96, (2018): 196–202.
21. Tähkämö, L., Partonen, T. and Pesonen, A. K., 'Systematic review of light exposure impact on human circadian rhythm.' *Chronobiology International*, 36(2), (2019): 151–70.
22. Kim, G. H., Kim, H. I., Paik, S. S. et al., 'Functional and morphological evalua-tion of blue light-emitting diode-induced retinal degeneration in mice.' *Graefe's Archive for Clinical and Experimental Ophthalmology*, 254(4), (2016): 705–16.
23. Geiger, P., Barben, M., Grimm, C. and Samardzija, M., 'Blue light-induced reti-nal lesions, intraretinal vascular leakage and edema formation in the all-cone mouse retina.' *Cell Death & Disease*, 6(11), (2015): e1985.
24. King, A., Gottlieb, E., Brooks, D. G. et al., 'Mitochondria-derived reactive oxygen species mediate blue light-induced death of retinal pigment epithelial cells.' *Photochemistry and Photobiology*, 79(5), (2004): 470–75.
25. Zhao, Z.-C., Zhou, Y., Tan, G. and Li, J., 'Research progress about the effect and prevention of blue light on eyes.' *International Journal of Ophthalmology*, 11(12), (2018): 1999–2003.
26. Vicente-Tejedor, J., Marchena, M., Ramírez, L. et al., 'Removal of the blue com-ponent of light significantly decreases retinal damage after high intensity exposure.' *PLoS One*, 13(3), (2018): e0194218.
27. Patra, V., Wagner, K., Arulampalam, V. and Wolf, P., 'Skin Microbiome Modu-lates the Effect of Ultraviolet Radiation on Cellular Response and Immune Function.' *iScience*, 15, (2019): 211–22.
28. Cicarma, E., Porojnicu, A. C., Lagunova, Z. et al., 'Sun and sun beds: inducers of vitamin D and skin cancer.' *Anticancer Research*, 29(9), (2009): 3495–500.
29. Garland, C.F., Garland, F. C., Gorham, E. D. et al., 'The role of vitamin D in cancer prevention.' *American Journal of Public Health*, 96(2), (2006): 252–61.
30. Rhodes, L. E., Webb, A. R., Fraser, H. I. et al., 'Recommended summer sunlight exposure levels can produce sufficient (> or =20 ng ml(−1)) but not the proposed optimal (> or =32 ng ml(−1)) 25(OH)D levels at UK latitudes.' *Journal of Investi-gative Dermatology*, 130(5), (2010): 1411–18.
31. Guzikowski J., Krzyścin J., Czerwińska A., Raszewska W., 'Adequate vitamin D$_3$ skin synthesis versus erythema risk in the Northern Hemisphere midlati-tudes.' J Photochem Photobiol B. 2018 Feb;179:54–65. doi: 10.1016/j.jphotobiol.2018.01.004. Epub 2018 Jan 11. PMID: 29334624.
32. An, S., Kim, K., Moon, S. et al., 'Indoor Tanning and the Risk of Overall and Early-Onset Melanoma and Non-Melanoma Skin Cancer: Systematic Review and Meta-Analysis.' *Cancers*, 13(23), (2021): 5940.
33. Webb, A. R., Kazantzidis, A., Kift, R.C. et al., 'Meeting Vitamin D Require-ments in White Caucasians at UK Latitudes: Providing a Choice.' *Nutrients*, 10(4), (2018): 497.
34. Clemens, T. L., Adams, J. S., Henderson, S. L. and Holick, M. F., 'Increased skin pigment reduces the capacity of skin to synthesise vitamin D3.' *The Lancet*, 1(8263), (1982): 74–6.
35. Mendes, M.M., Hart, K.H., Botelho, P.B. and Lanham-New, S., 'Vitamin D status in the tropics: Is sunlight exposure the main determinant?' *Nutrition Bulletin*, 43(4), (2018): 428–34.
36. Harinarayan, C. V., Holick, M. F., Prasad, U. V. et al., 'Vitamin D status and sun exposure in India.' *Dermato-Endocrinology*, 5(1), (2013): 130–41.

37. Wacker, M. and Holick, M. F., 'Sunlight and Vitamin D: A global perspective for health.' *Dermato-Endocrinology*, 5(1), (2013) :51–108.

38. Downs, C. A., Kramarsky-Winter, E., Fauth, J. E. et al., 'Toxicological effects of the sunscreen UV filter, benzophenone-2, on planulae and in vitro cells of the coral, *Stylophora pistillata*.' *Ecotoxicology*, 23(2), (2014): 175–91.

39. Downs, C. A., Kramarsky-Winter, E., Segal, R. et al., 'Toxicopathological Effects of the Sunscreen UV Filter, Oxybenzone (Benzophenone-3), on Coral Planulae and Cultured Primary Cells and Its Environmental Contamination in Hawaii and the U.S. Virgin Islands.' *Archives of Environmental Contamination and Toxicology*, 70(2), (2016): 265–88.

40. Thompson Coon, J., Boddy, K., Stein, K. et al., 'Does participating in physical activity in outdoor natural environments have a greater effect on physical and mental wellbeing than physical activity indoors? A systematic review.' *Environmental Science & Technology*, 45(5), (2011): 1761–72.

41. Bowler, D. E., Buyung-Ali, L. M., Knight, T. M. and Pullin, A. S., 'A systematic review of evidence for the added benefits to health of exposure to natural environments.' *BMC Public Health*, 10 (2010): 456.

42. Twohig-Bennett, C. and Jones, A., 'The health benefits of the great outdoors: A systematic review and meta-analysis of greenspace exposure and health outcomes.' *Environmental Research*, 166, (2018): 628–37.

43. Li, Q., Morimoto, K., Nakadai, A. et al., 'Forest bathing enhances human natural killer activity and expression of anti-cancer proteins.' *International Journal of Immunopathology and Pharmacology*, 20(2), (2007): 3–8.

44. Li, Q., Morimoto, K., Kobayashi, M. et al., 'A forest bathing trip increases human natural killer activity and expression of anti-cancer proteins in female subjects.' *Journal of Biological Regulators and Homeostatic Agents*, 22(1), (2008): 45–55.

45. Li, Q., Otsuka, T., Kobayashi, M. et al., 'Acute effects of walking in forest environments on cardiovascular and metabolic parameters.' *European Journal of Applied Physiology*, 111(11), (2011): 2845–53.

46. Ideno, Y., Hayashi, K., Abe, Y. et al., 'Blood pressure-lowering effect of *Shinrin-yoku* (Forest bathing): a systematic review and meta-analysis.' *BMC Complementary and Alternative Medicine*, 17(1), (2017): 409.

47. Park, B. J., Tsunetsugu, Y., Kasetani, T. et al., 'The physiological effects of *Shinrin-yoku* (taking in the forest atmosphere or forest bathing): evidence from field experiments in 24 forests across Japan.' *Environmental Health and Preventative Medicine*, 15(1), (2010): 18–26.

48. Focht, B. C., 'Brief walks in outdoor and laboratory environments: effects on affective responses, enjoyment, and intentions to walk for exercise.' *Research Quarterly for Exercise and Sport*, 80(3), (2009): 611–20.

49. World Health Organization, *Air Quality Guidelines: Global update 2005: Particulate matter, ozone, nitrogen dioxide and sulfur dioxide* (WHO Regional Office for Europe, 2006).

50. Office for Health Improvement and Disparities, 'Guidance: Air Pollution: applying All Our Health.' Updated 28 February 2022, https://www.gov.uk/government/publications/air-pollution-applying-all-our-health/air-pollution-applying-all-our-health

51. Zhang, J. and Smith, K. R., 'Indoor air pollution: a global health concern.' *British Medical Bulletin*, 68(1), (2003): 209–25.

52. Donlan, R. M., 'Biofilm Formation: A Clinically Relevant Microbiological Process.' *Clinical Infectious Diseases*, 33(8), Issue 8, 2001: 1387–92.

53. Cincinelli, A. and Martellini, T., 'Indoor Air Quality and Health.' *International Journal of Environmental Research and Public Health*, 14(11), (2017): 1286.

54. Haldar, K., George, L., Wang, Z. et al., 'The sputum microbiome is distinct between COPD and health, independent of smoking history.' *Respiratory Research*, 21(1), (2020): 183.

55. Tizek, L., Redlinger, E., Ring, J. et al., 'Urban vs rural – Prevalence of self-reported allergies in various occupational and regional settings.' *World Allergy Organization Journal*, 15(1), (2022): 100625.

56. Nichols, W. J., Blue Mind: Why Water Makes You Happier, more Connected and Better at What You Do (Little, Brown, 2014).

57. Gascon, M., Zijlema, W., Vert, C. et al., 'Outdoor blue spaces, human health and well-being: A systematic review of quantitative studies.' *International Journal of Hygiene and Environmental Health*, 220(8), (2017): 1207–21.

58. Cracknell, D., White, M., Pahl, S. et al., 'Marine Biota and Psychological Well-Being: A Preliminary Examination of Dose-Response Effects in an Aquarium Setting.' *Environment and Behavior*, 48(10), (2016): 1242–69.

59. Ihsan, M., Watson, G., Choo, H. C. et al., 'Skeletal Muscle Microvascular Adaptations Following Regular Cold Water Immersion.' *International Journal of Sports Medicine*, 41(2), (2020): 98–105.

60. Shevchuk, N. A., 'Adapted cold shower as a potential treatment for depression.' *Medical Hypotheses*, 70(5), (2008): 995–1001.

61. Kox, M., van Eijk, L. T., Zwaag, J. et al., 'Voluntary activation of the sympathetic nervous system and attenuation of the innate immune response in humans.' *Proceedings of the National Academy of Sciences of the United States of America*, 111(20), (20140: 7379–84.

62. Buijze, G. A., Sierevelt, I. N., van der Heijden, B. C. et al., 'The Effect of Cold Showering on Health and Work: A Randomized Controlled Trial.' *PLoS One*, 11(9), (2016): e0161749.

63. Menigoz, W., Latz, T. T., Ely, R. A. et al., 'Integrative and lifestyle medicine strategies should include Earthing (grounding): Review of research evidence and clinical observations.' *EXPLORE*, 16(3), (2020): 152–60.

64. Sokal, K. and Sokal, P., 'Earthing the Human Body Influences Physiologic Processes.' *The Journal of Alternative and Complementary Medicine*, 17(4), (2011): 301–8.

65. Lobo, V., Patil, A., Phatak, A. and Chandra, N., 'Free radicals, antioxidants and functional foods: Impact on human health.' *Pharmacognosy Reviews*, 4(8), (2010): 118–26.

66. Sinatra, S. T., Oschman, J. L., Chevalier, G. and Sinatra, D., 'Electric Nutrition: The Surprising Health and Healing Benefits of Biological Grounding (Earthing).' *Alternative Therapies in Health and Medicine*, 23(5), (2017): 8–16.

67. Brown, R., Chevalier, G. and Hill, M., 'Grounding after moderate eccentric contractions reduces muscle damage.' *Open Access Journal of Sports Medicine*, 6, (2015): 305–17.

68. Chevalier, G., Sinatra, S. T., Oschman, J. L. and Delany, R. M., 'Earthing (Grounding) the Human Body Reduces Blood Viscosity – A Major Factor in Cardiovascular Disease.' *The Journal of Alternative and Complementary Medicine*, 19(2), (2013): 102–10.

69. Chevalier, G., Sinatra, S. T., Oschman, J. L. et al., 'Earthing: health implications of reconnecting the human body to the Earth's surface electrons.' *Journal of Environmental and Public Health*, 2012, (2012): 291541.

70. Sokal, P. and Sokal, K., 'The neuromodulative role of earthing.' *Medical Hypotheses*, 77(5), (2011): 824–26.

71. van den Berg, M. M., Maas, J., Muller, R. et al., 'Autonomic Nervous System Responses to Viewing Green and Built Settings: Differentiating Between Sympathetic and Parasympathetic Activity.' *International Journal of Environmental Research and Public Health*, 12(12), (2015): 15860–74.

72. Ulrich, R. S., 'View through a window may influence recovery from surgery.' *Science*, 224(4647), (1984): 420–1.

73. Losa, G. A., 'The fractal geometry of life.' *Rivista di Biologia*, 102(1), (2009): 29–59.

74. Brown, D. K., Barton, J. L. and Gladwell, V. F., 'Viewing Nature Scenes Positively Affects Recovery of Autonomic Function Following Acute-Mental Stress.' *Environmental Science & Technology*, 47(11), (2013): 5562–69.

75. White, M. P., Pahl, S., Wheeler, B. W. et al., 'Natural environments and subjective wellbeing: Different types of exposure are associated with different aspects of wellbeing.' *Health Place*, 45, (2017): 77–84.

76. Wilson, E. O., *Biophilia* (Harvard University Press, 1984).

77. Gaekwad, J. S., Moslehian, A. S., Roös, P. B. and Walker, A., 'A Meta-Analysis of Emotional Evidence for the Biophilia Hypothesis and Implications for Biophilic Design.' *Frontiers in Psychology*, 13, (2022): 750245.

78. Twohig-Bennett, C. and Jones, A., 'The health benefits of the great outdoors: A systematic review and meta-analysis of greenspace exposure and health outcomes.' *Environmental Research*, 166, (2018): 628–37.

79. Grassini, S., 'A Systematic Review and Meta-Analysis of Nature Walk as an Intervention for Anxiety and Depression.' *Journal of Clinical Medicine*, 11(6), (2022): 1731.

80. Bratman, G. N., Hamilton, J. P., Hahn, K. S. et al., 'Nature experience reduces rumination and subgenual prefrontal cortex activation.' *Proceedings of the National Academy of Sciences of the United States of America*, 112(28), (2015): 8567–72.

81. Ryan, R. M., Weinstein, N., Bernstein, J. et al., 'Vitalizing effects of being outdoors and in nature.' *Journal of Environmental Psychology*, 30(2), (2010): 159–68.

82. James, P., Hart, J. E., Banay, R. F. and Laden, F., 'Exposure to Greenness and Mortality in a Nationwide Prospective Cohort Study of Women.' *Environmental Health Perspectives*, 124(9), (2016): 1344–52.

83. Leavell, M. A., Leiferman, J. A., Gascon, M. et al., 'Nature-Based Social Prescribing in Urban Settings to Improve Social Connectedness and Mental Well-being: A Review.' *Current Environmental Health Reports*, 6(4), (2019): 297–308.

84. Khan and Giurca et al., 'Social Prescribing Around the World: A World Map of Global Developments in Social Prescribing Across Different Health System Contexts' (Global Social Prescribing Alliance, World Health Organization and National Academy for Social Prescribing, 2023), https://socialprescribingacademy.org.uk/media/4lbdy5ip/social-prescribing-around-the-world.pdf.

85. Sabel, B. A., Wang, J., Cárdenas-Morales, L. et al., 'Mental stress as consequence and cause of vision loss: the dawn of psychosomatic ophthalmology for preventive and personalized medicine.' *EPMA Journal*, 9(2), (2018): 133–60.

86. Vanlessen, N., De Raedt, R., Koster, E. and Pourtois, G., 'Happy heart, smiling eyes: A systematic review of positive mood effects on broadening of visuospatial attention.' *Neuroscience and Biobehavioral Reviews*, 68, (2016): 816–37.

87. Jakhar, F., Rodrigues, G. R., Mendonca, T. M. et al., 'Dry eye symptoms and digital eyestrain – Emerging epidemics among university students due to online curriculum amid the COVID-19 pandemic. A cross-sectional study.' *Indian Journal of Ophthalmology*, 71(4), (2023): 1472–77.

88. Hartig, T. et al.,'Health Benefits of Nature Experience: Psychological, Social and Cultural Processes.' In Nilsson, K., Sangster, M., Gallis, C. et al. (eds.), *Forests, Trees and Human Health* (Springer Science, 2010).

89. Seymour, V., 'The Human–Nature Relationship and Its Impact on Health: A Critical Review.' *Frontiers in Public Health*, 4, (2016): 260.

90. World Health Organization, 'Household air pollution', 28 November 2022, https://www.who.int/news-room/fact-sheets/detail/household-air-pollution-and-health?gclid=EAIaIQobChMIwtaL2eazgQMVyfntCh0KWgG_EAAYASAAEgJsTvD_BwE.

91. Kim, S., Hong, S.-H., Bong, C.-K. and Cho, M.-H., 'Characterization of air freshener emission: the potential health effects.' *The Journal of Toxicological Sciences*, 40(5), (2015): 535–50.

92. Olin, A. C., Granung, G., Hagberg, S. et al., 'Respiratory health among bleachery workers exposed to ozone and chlorine dioxide.' *Scandinavian Journal of Work, Environment & Health*, 28(2), (2002): 117–23.

93. Matulonga, B., Rava, M., Siroux, V. et al., 'Women using bleach for home cleaning are at increased risk of non-allergic asthma.' *Respiratory Medicine*, 117, (2016): 264–71.

94. Casas, L., Espinosa, A., Borràs-Santos, A. et al., 'Domestic use of bleach and infections in children: a multicentre cross-sectional study.' *Occupational & Environmental Medicine*, 72(8), (2015): 602–4.

95. Loft, S., Andersen, Z. J., Jørgensen, J. T. et al., 'Use of candles and risk of cardiovascular and respiratory events in a Danish cohort study.' *Indoor Air*, 32(8), (2022): e13086.

96. Al Khathlan, N., Basuwaidan, M., Al Yami, S. et al., 'Extent of exposure to scented candles and prevalence of respiratory and non-respiratory symptoms amongst young university students.' *BMC Public Health*, 23(1), (2023): 80.

97. Zhang, Z., Tan, L., Huss, A. et al., 'Household incense burning and children's respiratory health: A cohort study in Hong Kong.' *Pediatric Pulmonology*, 54(4), (2019): 399–404.

98. Lin, T. C., Krishnaswamy, G. and Chi, D. S., 'Incense smoke: clinical, structural and molecular effects on airway disease.' *Clinical and Molecular Allergy*, 6, (2008): 3.

99. Mastrangelo, G., Fadda, E. and Marzia, V., 'Polycyclic aromatic hydrocarbons and cancer in man.' *Environmental Health Perspectives*, 104(11), (1996): 1166–70.

100. Wolverton, B. C., Douglas, W. L. and Bounds, K., 'A Study of Interior Landscape Plants for Indoor Air Pollution Abatement' (NASA, 1989). https://ntrs.nasa.gov/search.jsp?R=19930072988

101. Cummings, B. E. and Waring, M. S., 'Potted plants do not improve indoor air quality: a review and analysis of reported VOC removal efficiencies.' *Journal of Exposure Science & Environmental Epidemiology*, 30(2), (2020): 253–61.

102. Lee, M. S., Lee, J., Park, B. J. and Miyazaki, Y., 'Interaction with indoor plants may reduce psychological and physiological stress by suppressing autonomic nervous system activity in young adults: a randomized crossover study.' *Journal of Physiology Anthropology*, 34(1), (2015): 21.

103. Han, K.-T., Ruan, L.-W. and Liao, L.-S., 'Effects of Indoor Plants on Human Functions: A Systematic Review with Meta-Analyses.' *International Journal of Environmental Research and Public Health*, 19(12), (2022): 7454.

104. Nieuwenhuis, M., Knight, C., Postmes, T. and Haslam, S. A., 'The relative benefits of green versus lean office space: three field experiments.' *Journal of Experimental Psychology Applied*, 20(3), (2014): 199–214.

105. Han, K. T. and Ruan, L. W., 'Effects of indoor plants on air quality: a systematic review.' *Environmental Science and Pollution Research*, 27(14), (2020): 16019–51.

106. Konieczna, A., Rutkowska, A. and Rachoń, D., 'Health risk of exposure to Bisphenol A (BPA).' *Rocz Panstw Zakl Hig*, 66(1), (2015): 5–11.

107. Fenichel, P., Chevalier, N. and Brucker-Davis, F., 'Bisphenol A: an endocrine and metabolic disruptor.' *Annales d'Endocrinologie*, 74(3), (2013): 211–20.

108. Sajid, M. and Ilyas, M., 'PTFE-coated non-stick cookware and toxicity concerns: a perspective.' *Environmental Science and Pollution Research*, 24(30), (2017): 23436–40.

109. Gaber, N., Bero, L. and Woodruff, T. J., 'The Devil they Knew: Chemical Documents Analysis of Industry Influence on PFAS Science.' *Annals of Global Health*, 89(1), (2023): 37.

110. Weatherly, L. M. and Gosse, J. A., 'Triclosan Exposure, Transformation, and Human Health Effects.' *Journal of Toxicology and Environmental Health – Part B: Critical Reviews*, 20(8), (2017): 447–69.

111. Balwierz, R., Biernat, P., Jasińska-Balwierz, A. et al., 'Potential Carcinogens in Makeup Cosmetics.' *International Journal of Environmental Research and Public Health*, 20(6), (2023): 4780.

112. Kwon, Y., 'Assessing an Overall Toxicological Implication of Nail Care Product for Occupational and Consumer Health Improvement.' *Iranian Journal of Public Health*, 51(5), (2022): 1185–87.

113. Gao, C.-J. and Kannan, K., 'Phthalates, bisphenols, parabens, and triclocarban in feminine hygiene products from the United States and their implications for human exposure.' *Environment International*, 136, (2020): 105465.

114. Vethaak, A. D. and Legler, J., 'Microplastics and human health.' *Science*, 371(6530), (2021): 672–4.

115. Hernandez, L. M., Xu, E. G., Larsson, H. C. E. et al., 'Plastic Teabags Release Billions of Microparticles and Nanoparticles into Tea.' *Environmental Science & Technology*, 53(21), (2019): 12300–10.

116. Wang, Y. and Qian, H., 'Phthalates and Their Impacts on Human Health.' *Healthcare*, 9(5), (2021): 603.

117. Diamanti-Kandarakis, E., Bourguignon, J. P., Giudice, L. C. et al., 'Endocrine-Disrupting Chemicals: An Endocrine Society Scientific Statement.' *Endocrine Reviews*, 30(4), (2009): 293–342.

118. Xu, J., Ye, Y., Huang, F. et al., 'Association between dioxin and cancer incidence and mortality: a meta-analysis.' *Scientific Reports*, 6, (2016): 38012.

119. Ahern, T. P., Broe, A., Lash, T. L. et al., 'Phthalate Exposure and Breast Cancer Incidence: A Danish Nationwide Cohort Study.' *Journal of Clinical Oncology*, 37(21), (2019): 1800–9.

120. Roeleveld, N. and Bretveld, R., 'The impact of pesticides on male fertility.' *Current Opinion in Obstetrics and Gynecology*, 20(3), (2008): 229–33.

121. Bustamante-Montes, L. P., Hernández-Valero, M. A., Flores-Pimentel, D. et al., 'Prenatal exposure to phthalates is associated with decreased anogenital distance

and penile size in male newborns.' *Journal of Developmental Origins of Health and Disease*, 4(4), (2013): 300–6.

122. Gambino, I., Bagordo, F., Grassi, T. et al., 'Occurrence of Microplastics in Tap and Bottled Water: Current Knowledge.' *International Journal of Environmental Research and Public Health*, 19(9), (2022): 5283.

123. Danailova, Y., Velikova, T., Nikolaev, G. et al., 'Nutritional Management of Thyroiditis of Hashimoto.' *International Journal of Molecular Sciences*, 23(9), (2022): 5144.

Vegetables

1. Newman, G., *The Plant Power Doctor: A simple prescription for a healthier you* (Ebury Press, 2021).

2. Kim, H., Caulfield, L. E., Garcia-Larsen, V. et al., 'Plant-Based Diets Are Associated With a Lower Risk of Incident Cardiovascular Disease, Cardiovascular Disease Mortality, and All-Cause Mortality in a General Population of Middle-Aged Adults.' *Journal of American Heart Association*, 8(16), (2019): e012865.

3. Kim, H., Caulfield, L E. and Rebholz, C. M., 'Healthy Plant-Based Diets Are Associated with Lower Risk of All-Cause Mortality in US Adults.' *The Journal of Nutrition*, 148(4), (2018): 624–31.

4. Turner-McGrievy, G. M., Wirth, M. D., Shivappa, N. et al., 'Randomization to plant-based dietary approaches leads to larger short-term improvements in Dietary Inflammatory Index scores and macronutrient intake compared with diets that contain meat.' *Nutrition Research*, 35(2), (2015): 97–106.

5. Kim, M. K., Cho, S. W. and Park, Y. K., 'Long-term vegetarians have low oxidative stress, body fat, and cholesterol levels.' *Nutrition Research and Practice*, 6(2), (2012): 155–61.

6. Liu, R. H., 'Health benefits of fruit and vegetables are from additive and synergistic combinations of phytochemicals.' *The American Journal of Clinical Nutrition*, 78(3), (2003): 517S–520S.

7. Chiavaroli, L., Nishi, S. K., Khan, T. A. et al., 'Portfolio Dietary Pattern and Cardiovascular Disease: A Systematic Review and Meta-analysis of Controlled Trials.' *Progress in Cardiovascular Diseases*, 61(1), (2018): 43–53.

8. Chiavaroli, L., Viguiliouk, E., Nishi, S. K. et al., 'DASH Dietary Pattern and Cardiometabolic Outcomes: An Umbrella Review of Systematic Reviews and Meta-Analyses.' *Nutrients*, 11(2), (2019): 338.

9. Viguiliouk, E., Glenn, A. J., Nishi, S. K. et al., 'Associations Between Dietary Pulses Alone or with Other Legumes and Cardiometabolic Disease Outcomes: An Umbrella Review and Updated Systematic Review and Meta-analysis of Prospective Cohort Studies.' *Advances in Nutrition*, 10(suppl. 4): S308–19.

10. Viguiliouk, E., Kendall, C. W., Kahleová, H. et al., 'Effect of vegetarian dietary patterns on cardiometabolic risk factors in diabetes: A systematic review and meta-analysis of randomized controlled trials.' *Clinical Nutrition*, 38(3), (2019): 1133–45.

11. Katz, D. L., Frates, E. P., Bonnet, J. P. et al., 'Lifestyle as Medicine: The Case for a True Health Initiative.' *American Journal of Health Promotion*, 32(6), (2018): 1452–58.

12. GBD 2017 Diet Collaborators, 'Health effects of dietary risks in 195 countries, 1990–2017: a systematic analysis for the Global Burden of Disease Study 2017.' *The Lancet*, 393(10184), (2019): 1958–72.

13. Li, Y., Pan, A., Wang, D. D. et al., 'Impact of Healthy Lifestyle Factors on Life Expectancies in the US Population.' *Circulation*, 138, (2018): 345–55.

14. Kvaavik, E., Batty, D., Ursin, G. et al., 'Influence of Individual and Combined Health Behaviours on Total and Cause-Specific Mortality in Men and Women: The United Kingdom Health and Lifestyle Survey', *Archives of Internal Medicine*, 170(8), (2010): 711–18.

15. Rose, S. and Strombom, A., 'Breast Cancer Prevention with a Plant-Based Diet.' *Cancer Therapy & Oncology International Journal*, 17(1), (2020): 555955.

16. Rose, S. and Strombom, A., 'Stomach Cancer – Prevention with a Plant-Based Diet.' *Cancer Therapy & Oncology International Journal*, 19(3), (2021): 556012.

17. Chen, Z., Wang, P. P., Woodrow, J. et al., 'Dietary patterns and colorectal cancer: results from a Canadian population-based study.' *Nutrition Journal*, 14, (2015): 8.

18. Lanou, A. J. and Svenson, B., 'Reduced cancer risk in vegetarians: an analysis of recent reports.' *Cancer Management and Research*, 3, (2011): 1–8.

19. Sandhu, M., White, I. R. and McPherson, K., 'Systematic review of the prospective cohort studies on meat consumption and colorectal cancer risk: a meta-analytical approach.' *Cancer Epidemiology, Biomarkers & Prevention*, 10(5), (2001): 439–46.

20. Giovannucci, E., Rimm, E. B., Colditz, G. A. et al., 'A prospective study of dietary fat and risk of prostate cancer.' *Journal of National Cancer Institute*, 85(19), (1993): 1571–9.

21. Le Marchand, L., Kolonel, L., Wilkens, L. R. et al., 'Animal fat consumption and prostate cancer: a prospective study in Hawaii.' *Epidemiology*, 5(3), (1994): 276–82.

22. Sathiaraj, E., Afshan, K., Sruthi, R. et al., 'Effects of a Plant-Based High-Protein Diet on Fatigue in Breast Cancer Patients Undergoing Adjuvant Chemotherapy – a Randomized Controlled Trial.' *Nutrition and Cancer*, 75(3), (2023): 846–56.

23. Sandefur, K., Kahleova, H., Desmond, A. N. et al., 'Crohn's Disease Remission with a Plant-Based Diet: A Case Report.' *Nutrients*, 11(6), (20190: 1385.

24. Chiba, M., Nakane, K., Tsuji, T. et al., 'Relapse Prevention in Ulcerative Colitis by Plant-Based Diet Through Educational Hospitalization: A Single-Group Trial.' *The Permanente Journal*, 22 (3), (2018): 17–167.

25. McMacken, M. and Shah, S., 'A plant-based diet for the prevention and treatment of type 2 diabetes.' *Journal of Geriatric Cardiology*, 14(5), (2017): 342–54.

26. Rizzo, N., Sabaté, J., Jaceldo-Siegl, K. and Fraser, G. E., 'Vegetarian dietary patterns are associated with a lower risk of metabolic syndrome: the adventist health study 2.' *Diabetes Care*, 34(5), (2011): 1225–7.

27. Rose, S. and Strombom, A., 'Lupus – Prevention and Treatment with a Plant-Based Diet.' *Orthopedics & Rheumatology*, 21(1), (2023): 556060.

28. Kutlu, A., Oztürk, S., Taşkapan, O. et al., 'Meat-induced joint attacks, or meat attacks the joint: rheumatism versus allergy.' *Nutrition in Clinical Practice*, 25(1), (2010): 90–1.

29. Müller, H., de Toledo, F. W. and Resch, K. L., 'Fasting followed by vegetarian diet in patients with rheumatoid arthritis: a systematic review.' *Scandinavian Journal of Rheumatology*, 30(1), (2001): 1–10.

30. McDougall, J., Bruce, B., Spiller, G. et al., 'Effects of a very low-fat, vegan diet in subjects with rheumatoid arthritis.' *The Journal of Alternative and Complementary Medicine*, 8(1), (2002): 71–5.

31. Barnard, N. D., Holtz, D. N., Schmidt, N., et al., 'Nutrition in the prevention and treatment of endometriosis: A review.' *Frontiers in Nutrition*, 10, (2023).

32. Barnard, N. D., Scialli, A. R., Hurlock, D. and Bertron, P., 'Diet and sex-hormone binding globulin, dysmenorrhea, and premenstrual symptoms.' *Obstetrics & Gynecology*, 95(2), (2000): 245–50.

33. Shen, Y., Wu, Y., Lu, Q. and Ren, M., 'Vegetarian diet and reduced uterine fibroids risk: A case-control study in Nanjing, China.' *The Journal of Obstetrics and Gynaecology Research*, 42(1), (2016): 87–94.

34. Barnard, N. D., Kahleova, H., Holtz, D. N. et al., 'The Women's Study for the Alleviation of Vasomotor Symptoms (WAVS): a randomized, controlled trial of a plant-based diet and whole soybeans for postmenopausal women.' *Menopause*, 28(10), (2021): 1150–56.

35. Klementova, M., Thieme, L., Haluzik, M. et al., 'A Plant-Based Meal Increases Gastrointestinal Hormones and Satiety More Than an Energy- and Macronutrient-Matched Processed-Meat Meal in T2D, Obese, and Healthy Men: A Three-Group Randomized Crossover Study.' *Nutrients*, 11(1), (2019): 157.

36. Crowe, F. L., Appleby, P. N., Allen, N. E. and Key, T. J., 'Diet and risk of diverticular disease in Oxford cohort of European Prospective Investigation into Cancer and Nutrition (EPIC): prospective study of British vegetarians and non-vegetarians.' *The BMJ*, 343, (2011).

37. Rose, S. and Strombom, A., 'Preventing Thyroid Diseases with a Plant-Based Diet, While Ensuring Adequate Iodine Status.' *Global Journal of Otolaryngology*, 21(4), (2020): 556069.

38. Harirchian, M. H., Karimi, E. and Bitarafan, S., 'Diet and disease-related outcomes in multiple sclerosis: A systematic review of clinical trials.' *Current Journal of Neurology*, 21(1), (2022): 52–63.

39. Yadav, V., Marracci, G., Kim, E. et al., 'Low-fat, plant-based diet in multiple sclerosis: A randomized controlled trial.' *Multiple Sclerosis and Related Disorders*, 9, (2016): 80–90.

40. Fusano, M., 'Veganism in acne, atopic dermatitis, and psoriasis: Benefits of a plant-based diet.' *Clinics in Dermatology*, 41(1), (2023): 122–6.

41. Fam, V. W., Charoenwoodhipong, P., Sivamani, R. K. et al., 'Plant-Based Foods for Skin Health: A Narrative Review.' *Journal of the Academy of Nutrition and Dietetics*, 122(3), (2022): 614–29.

42. Lewandowska, M., Dunbar, K. and Kassam, S., 'Managing Psoriatic Arthritis With a Whole Food Plant-Based Diet: A Case Study.' *American Journal of Lifestyle Medicine*, 15(4), (2021): 402–6.

43. Khalid, W., Arshad, M. S., Ranjha, M. M. A. N. et al., 'Functional constituents of plant-based foods boost immunity against acute and chronic disorders.' *Open Life Sciences*, 17(1), (2022): 1075–93.

44. Jiang, L., Zhang, G., Li, Y. et al., 'Potential Application of Plant-Based Functional Foods in the Development of Immune Boosters.' *Frontiers in Pharmacology*, 12, (2021): 637782.

45. Wong, C. S., Lim, C. W., Mohammed, H. I. et al., 'Current Perspective of Plant-Based Diets on Communicable Diseases Caused by Viruses: A Mini Review.' *Frontiers in Nutrition*, 9, (2022): 786972.

46. IPCC, 'AR6 Synthesis Report: Climate Change 2023'. A report of the Intergovernmental Panel on Climate Change finalised during the panel's 58th session held in Interlaken, Switzerland, 13–19 March 2023. https://www.ipcc.ch/report/sixth-assessment-report-cycle/

47. Martin, M. J., Thottathil, S. E. and Newman, T. B., 'Antibiotics Overuse in Animal Agriculture: A Call to Action for Health Care Providers.' *American Journal of Public Health*, 105(12), (2015): 2409–10.

48. O'Neill, J., *Antimicrobial Resistance: Tackling a crisis for the health and wealth of nations* (Review on Antimicrobial Resistance, 2014).

49. United Nations Interagency Coordination Group on Antimicrobial Resistance, 'No Time to Wait: Securing the future from drug-resistant infections', 29 April 2019, https://www.who.int/publications/i/item/no-time-to-wait-securing-the-future-from-drug-resistant-infections.

50. Sala, E., Mayorga, J., Bradley, D. et al., 'Protecting the global ocean for biodiversity, food and climate.' *Nature*, 592, (2021): 397–402.

51. https://www.plasticatbay.org/marine-scotlands-marine-litter-strategy-2022-consultation-plasticbay-response/?v=79cba1185463

52. Lebreton, L., Slat, B., Ferrari, F. et al., 'Evidence that the Great Pacific Garbage Patch is rapidly accumulating plastic.' *Scientific Reports*, 8, (2018): 4666.

53. Enyoh, C. E., Verla, A. W., Verla, E. N. et al., 'Airborne microplastics: a review study on method for analysis, occurrence, movement and risks.' *Environmental Monitoring Assessment*, 191(11), (2019): 668.

54. Marcelino, R. C., Cardoso, R. M., Domingues, E. L. B. C. et al, 'The emerging risk of microplastics and nanoplastics on the microstructure and function of reproductive organs in mammals: A systematic review of preclinical evidence.' *Life Sciences*, 295, (2022): 120404.

55. Ragusa, A., Matta, M., Cristiano, L. et al., 'Deeply in Plasticenta: Presence of Microplastics in the Intracellular Compartment of Human Placentas.' *International Journal of Environmental Research and Public Health*, 19(18), (2022): 11593.

56. UNICEF, *The Climate Crisis is a Child Rights Crisis: Introducing the Children's Climate Risk Index*. (UNICEF, 2021).

57. Prillaman, M., 'Are we in the Anthropocene? Geologists could define new epoch for Earth.' *Nature*, 613(7942), (2023): 14–15.

58. Willett, W., Rockström, J., Loken, B. et al., 'Food in the Anthropocene: the EAT-Lancet Commission on healthy diets from sustainable food systems.' *The Lancet*, 393(10170), (2019): 447–92.

59. Firth, J., Marx, W., Dash, S. et al., 'The Effects of Dietary Improvement on Symptoms of Depression and Anxiety: A Meta-Analysis of Randomized Controlled Trials.' *Psychosomatic Medicine*, 81(3), (2019): 265–80.

60. Jacka, F. N., O'Neil, A., Opie, R. et al., 'A randomised controlled trial of dietary improvement for adults with major depression (the "SMILES" trial).' *BMC Medicine*, 15(1), (2017): 23.

61. Agarwal, U., Mishra, S., Xu, J. et al., 'A multicenter randomized controlled trial of a nutrition intervention program in a multiethnic adult population in the corporate setting reduces depression and anxiety and improves quality of life: the GEICO study.' *American Journal of Health Promotion*, 29(4), (20150: 245–54.

62. Zhang, L., Chen, T., Yin, Y. et al., 'Dietary microRNA – A Novel Functional Component of Food.' *Advances in Nutrition*, 10(4), (2019): 711–21.

63. Wiertsema, S. P., van Bergenhenegouwen, J., Garssen, J. et al., 'The Interplay between the Gut Microbiome and the Immune System in the Context of Infectious Diseases throughout Life and the Role of Nutrition in Optimizing Treatment Strategies.' *Nutrients*, 13(3), (2021): 886.

64. D'Acquisto, F., 'Affective immunology: where emotions and the immune response converge.' *Dialogues in Clinical Neuroscience*, 19(1), (2017): 9–19.

65. Masih, J., Belschak, F. et al., 'Mood configurations and their relationship to immune system responses: Exploring the relationship between moods, immune system responses, thyroid hormones, and social support.' *PLoS One*, 14(5), (2019): e0216232.

66. Kovats, S., 'Estrogen receptors regulate innate immune cells and signaling pathways.' *Cellular Immunology*, 294(2), (2015): 63–9.

67. Rifé, S. U., Márquez, M. G., Escalante, A. and Velich, T., 'The effect of testosterone on the immune response. 1. Mechanism of action on antibody-forming cells.' *Immunological Investment*, 19(3), (1990): 259–70.

68. Fung, T. C., Olson, C. A. and Hsiao, E. Y., 'Interactions between the microbiota, immune and nervous systems in health and disease.' *Nature Neuroscience*, 20(2), (2017): 145–55.Chang, H. H. and Chen, P. S., 'Inflammatory Biomarkers for Mood Disorders - A Brief Narrative Review.' *Current Pharmaceutical Design*, 26(2), (2020): 236–43.

69. Rosenblat, J. D., Cha, D. S., Mansur, R. B. and McIntyre, R. S., 'Inflamed moods: a review of the interactions between inflammation and mood disorders.' *Progress in Neuro-psychopharmacoloy and Biological Psychiatry*, 53, (2014): 23–34.

70. Khan, W. I. and Ghia, J. E., 'Gut hormones: emerging role in immune activation and inflammation.' *Clinical & Experimental Immunology*, 161(1), (2010): 19–27.

71. Forsyth, C. B., Shannon, K. M., Kordower, J. H. et al., 'Increased intestinal permeability correlates with sigmoid mucosa alpha-synuclein staining and endotoxin exposure markers in early Parkinson's disease.' *PLoS One*, 6(12), (2011): e28032.

72. André, P., Laugerette, F. and Féart, C., 'Metabolic Endotoxemia: A Potential Underlying Mechanism of the Relationship between Dietary Fat Intake and Risk for Cognitive Impairments in Humans?' *Nutrients*, 11(8), (2019): 1887.

73. Pendyala, S., Walker, J. M. and Holt, P. R., 'A high-fat diet is associated with endotoxemia that originates from the gut.' *Gastroenterology*, 142(5), (2012): 1100–1.

74. Zhao, T., Wei, Y., Zhu, Y. et al., 'Gut microbiota and rheumatoid arthritis: From pathogenesis to novel therapeutic opportunities.' *Frontiers in Immunology*, 13, (2022): 1007165.

75. Lee, J. W., Lee, Y. K., Yuk, D. Y. et al., 'Neuro-inflammation induced by lipopolysaccharide causes cognitive impairment through enhancement of beta-amyloid generation.' *Journal of Neuroinflammation*, 5, (2008): 37.

76. Cerovic, M., Forloni, G. and Balducci, C., 'Neuroinflammation and the Gut Microbiota: Possible Alternative Therapeutic Targets to Counteract Alzheimer's Disease?' *Frontiers in Aging Neuroscience*, 11, (2019): 284.

77. Desai, M. S., Seekatz, A. M., Koropatkin, N. M. et al., 'A Dietary Fiber-Deprived Gut Microbiota Degrades the Colonic Mucus Barrier and Enhances Pathogen Susceptibility.' *Cell*, 167(5), (2016): 1339–53.

78. Silva, Y. P., Bernardi, A., Frozza, R. L., 'The Role of Short-Chain Fatty Acids From Gut Microbiota in Gut-Brain Communication.' *Frontiers in Endocrinology*, 11, (2020): 25.

79. Xiong, R. G., Zhou, D. D., Wu, S.-X. et al., 'Health Benefits and Side Effects of Short-Chain Fatty Acids.' *Foods*, 11(18), (2022): 2863.

80. Müller, B., Rasmusson, A. J., Just, D. et al., 'Fecal Short-Chain Fatty Acid Ratios as Related to Gastrointestinal and Depressive Symptoms in Young Adults.' *Psychosomatic Medicine*, 83(7), (2021): 693–99.

81. Wenzel, T. J., Gates, E. J., Ranger, A. L. and Klegeris, A., 'Short-chain fatty acids (SCFAs) alone or in combination regulate select immune functions of microglia-like cells.' *Molecular and Cellular Neuroscience*, 105, (2020): 103493.

82. Fock, E. and Parnova, R., 'Mechanisms of Blood–Brain Barrier Protection by Microbiota-Derived Short-Chain Fatty Acids.' *Cells*, 12(4), (2023): 657.

83. Knowles, S. R., Nelson, E. A. and Palombo, E. A., 'Investigating the role of perceived stress on bacterial flora activity and salivary cortisol secretion: a possible mechanism underlying susceptibility to illness.' *Biological Psychology*, 77(2), (2008): 132–7.

84. Alkasir, R., Li, J., Li, X. et al., 'Human gut microbiota: the links with dementia development.' *Protein Cell*, 8(2), (2017): 90–102.

85. Folstein, M., Liu, T., Peter, I. et al., 'The homocysteine hypothesis of depression.' *American Journal of Psychiatry*, 164(6), (2007): 861–7.

86. Tsai, A. C., Chang, T.-L., Chi, S.-H., 'Frequent consumption of vegetables predicts lower risk of depression in older Taiwanese – results of a prospective population based study.' *Public Health Nutrition*, 15(6), (2012): 1087–92.

87. Tolmunen, T., Hintikka, J., Ruusunen, A. et al., 'Dietary folate and the risk of depression in Finnish middle-aged men. A prospective follow up study.' *Psychotherapy and Psychosomatics*, 73(6), (2004): 334–9.

88. Beydoun, M. A., Beydoun, H. A., Boueiz, A. et al., 'Antioxidant status and its association with elevated depressive symptoms among US adults. National Health and Nutrition Examination Surveys 2005–6.' *British Journal of Nutrition*, 109(9), (2013): 1714–29.

89. Guo, X., Park, Y., Freedman, N. D. et al., 'Sweetened beverages, coffee, and tea and depression risk among older US adults.' *PLos One*, 9(4), (2014): e94715.

90. Walton, R. G., Hudak, R. and Green-Waite, R. J., 'Adverse reactions to aspartame: double-blind challenge in patients from a vulnerable population.' *Biological Psychiatry*, 34(1-2), (1993): 13–17.

91. Tsai, J.-H., Huang, C.-F., Lin, M.-N. et al., 'Taiwanese Vegetarians Are Associated with Lower Dementia Risk: A Prospective Cohort Study.' *Nutrients*, 14(3), (2022): 588.

92. Farvid, M. S., Ding, M., Pan, A. et al., 'Dietary linoleic acid and risk of coronary heart disease: a systematic review and meta-analysis of prospective cohort studies.' *Circulation*, 130(18), (2014): 1568–78.

93. Li, J., Guasch-Ferré, M., Li, Y. and Hu, F. B., 'Dietary intake and biomarkers of linoleic acid and mortality: systematic review and meta-analysis of prospective cohort studies.' *The American Journal of Clinical Nutrition*, 112(1), (2020): 150–67.

94. Esselstyn, C. B., 'A plant-based diet and coronary artery disease: a mandate for effective therapy.' *Journal of Geriatric Cardiology*, 14(5), (2017): 317–20.

95. Voigt, R. M., Forsyth, C. B., Green, S. J. et al., 'Circadian Rhythm and the Gut Microbiome.' *International Review of Neurobiology*, 131, (2016): 193–205.

96. Rehm, J., 'The Risks Associated With Alcohol Use and Alcoholism.' *Alcohol Research & Health*, 34(2), (2011): 135–43.

97. Kushner, M. G., Abrams, K. and Borchardt, C., 'The relationship between anxiety disorders and alcohol use disorders: a review of major perspectives and findings.' *Clinical Psychology Review*, 20(2), (2000): 149–71.

98. Thakkar, M. M., Sharma, R. and Sahota, P., 'Alcohol disrupts sleep homeostasis.' *Alcohol*, 49(4), (2015): 299–310.

99. D'Silva, A., Marshall, D. A., Vallance, J. K. et al., 'Meditation and Yoga for Irritable Bowel Syndrome: A Randomized Clinical Trial.' *The American Journal of Gastroenterology*, 118(2), (2023): 329–37.

100. Glynn, H., Möller, S. P., Wilding, H. et al., 'Prevalence and Impact of Post-traumatic Stress Disorder in Gastrointestinal Conditions: A Systematic Review.' *Digestive Diseases and Sciences*, 66(12), (2021): 4109–19.

101. Wong, W. M., 'Restriction of FODMAP in the management of bloating in irritable bowel syndrome.' *Singapore Medical Journal*, 57(9), (2016): 476–84.

102. Bulsiewicz, W. with recipes by Caspero, A., *The Fibre Fuelled Cookbook: Inspiring Plant-based Recipes to Turbocharge Your Health* (Vermilion, 2022).

103. Sinha, R., 'Role of addiction and stress neurobiology on food intake and obesity.' *Biological Psychology*, 131, (2018): 5–13. (Please note: Dr Sinha is on the Scientific Advisory Board for Embera NeuroTherapeutics, Inc.)

104. Tonstad, S., Stewart, K., Oda, K. et al., 'Vegetarian diets and incidence of diabetes in the Adventist Health Study-2.' *Nutrition, Metabolism & Cardiovascular Diseases*, 23(4), (2013): 292–9.

105. Watling, C. Z., Schmidt, J. A., Dunneram, Y. et al., 'Risk of cancer in regular and low meat-eaters, fish-eaters, and vegetarians: a prospective analysis of UK Biobank participants.' *BMC Medicine*, 20(1), (2022): 73.

106. Ferguson, J. J., Oldmeadow, C., Mishra, G. D. and Garg, M. L., 'Plant-based dietary patterns are associated with lower body weight, BMI and waist circumference in older Australian women.' *Public Health Nutrition*, 25(1), (2022): 18–31.

107. Lindeman, M., Stark, K. and Latvala, K., 'Vegetarianism and Eating-Disordered Thinking.' *Eating Disorders*, 8(2), (2000): 157–65.

108. Baş M., Karabudak, E. and Kiziltan, G., 'Vegetarianism and eating disorders: association between eating attitudes and other psychological factors among Turkish adolescents.' *Appetite*, 44(3), (2005): 309–15.

109. Klopp, S. A., Heiss, C. J. and Smith, H. S., 'Self-reported vegetarianism may be a marker for college women at risk for disordered eating.' *Journal of the Academy of Nutrition and Dietetics*, 103(6), (2003): 745–47.

110. Neumark-Sztainer, D., Story, M., Resnick, M. D. and Blum, R. W., 'Adolescent vegetarians. A behavioral profile of a school-based population in Minnesota.' *The Archives of Pediatrics & Adolescent Medicine*, 151(8), (1997): 833–38.

111. Robinson-O'Brien, R., Perry, C. L., Wall, M. M. et al., 'Adolescent and young adult vegetarianism: better dietary intake and weight outcomes but increased risk of disordered eating behaviors.' *Journal of the Academy of Nutrition and Dietetics*, 109(4), (2009): 648–55.

112. Bardone-Cone, A. M., Fitzsimmons-Craft, E. E., Harney, M. B. et al., 'The inter-relationships between vegetarianism and eating disorders among females.' *Journal of the Academy of Nutrition and Dietetics*, 112(8), (2012): 1247–52.

113. Amit, M., 'Vegetarian diets in children and adolescents.' *Paediatrics and Child Health*, 15(5), (2010): 303–14.

114. O'Connor, M. A., Touyz, S. W., Dunn, S. M. and Beumont, P. J., 'Vegetarianism in anorexia nervosa? A review of 116 consecutive cases.' *The Medical Journal of Australia*, 147(11-12), (1987): 540–2.

115. Forestell, C. A., Spaeth, A. M. and Kane, S. A., 'To eat or not to eat red meat. A closer look at the relationship between restrained eating and vegetarianism in college females.' *Appetite*, 58(1), (2012): 319–25.

116. Timko, C. A., Hormes, J. M. and Chubski, J., 'Will the real vegetarian please stand up? An investigation of dietary restraint and eating disorder symptoms in vegetarians versus non-vegetarians.' *Appetite*, 58(3), (2012): 982–90.

117. Heiss, S., Coffino, J. A. and Hormes, J. M., 'Eating and health behaviors in vegans compared to omnivores: Dispelling common myths.' *Appetite*, 118, (2017): 129–35.

118. Maclean, P. S., Bergouignan, A., Cornier, M. A. and Jackman, M. R., 'Biology's response to dieting: the impetus for weight regain.' *American Journal of Physiology – Regulatory, Integrative and Comparative Physiology*, 301(3), (2011): R581–600.

119. Mann, T., Tomiyama, A. J., Westling, E. et al., 'Medicare's search for effective obesity treatments: diets are not the answer.' *American psychologist*, 62(3), (2007): 220–33.

120. Anderson, J. W., Konz, E. C., Frederich, R. C. and Wood, C. L., 'Long-term weight-loss maintenance: a meta-analysis of US studies.' *The American Journal of Clinical Nutrition*, 74(5), (2001): 579–84.

121. Sumithran, P., Prendergast, L. A., Delbridge, E. et al., 'Long-term persistence of hormonal adaptations to weight loss.' *The New England Journal of Medicine*, 365(17), (2011): 1597–604.

122. Polidori, D., Sanghvi, A., Seeley, R. J. and Hall, K. D., 'How Strongly Does Appetite Counter Weight Loss? Quantification of the Feedback Control of Human Energy Intake.' *Obesity (Silver Spring)*, 24(11), (2016): 2289–95.

123. Hall, K. D. and Kahan, S., 'Maintenance of lost weight and long-term management of obesity.' *Medical Clinics of North America*, 102(1), (2018): 183–97.

124. Hazzard, V. M., Loth, K. A., Crosby, R. D. et al., 'Relative food abundance predicts greater binge-eating symptoms in subsequent hours among young adults experiencing food insecurity: Support for the "feast-or-famine" cycle hypothesis from an ecological momentary assessment study.' *Appetite*, 180, (2023): 106316.

125. Wise, J., 'Britain's deprived areas have five times as many fast food shops as rich areas.' *BMJ*, 363, (2018): k4661.

126. The Trussell Trust, 'End of Year Stats', https://www.trusselltrust.org/news-and-blog/latest-stats/end-year-stats/.

127. Wiss, D. A. and Brewerton, T. D., 'Adverse Childhood Experiences and Adult Obesity: A Systematic Review of Plausible Mechanisms and Meta-Analysis of Cross-Sectional Studies,' *Physiology & Behavior*, 223, (2020): 112964.

128. McAleavey, K., 'Ten years of treating eating disorders: what have we learned? A personal perspective on the application of 12-step and wellness programs.' *Advances in Mind–Body Medicine*, 23(2), (2008): 18–26.

129. Freire, R., 'Scientific evidence of diets for weight loss: Different macronutrient composition, intermittent fasting, and popular diets.' *Nutrition*, 69, (2020): 110549.

130. Kemp, T., Lopez, N. V., Ward, S., Sherzai, D., Sherzai, A. and Sutliffe, J., 'The INFINITE Study: Pilot Research Exploring Plant-Based Nutrition in Treatment for Substance Use Disorders.' *American Journal of Lifestyle Medicine*, (2022).

Exercise

1. Zhang, Z., Chen, W., 'A Systematic Review of the Relationship Between Physical Activity and Happiness.' *Journal of Happiness Studies*, 20(4), (2019): 1305–22.
2. Schuch, F. B., Vancampfort, D., Richards, J. et al., 'Exercise as a treatment for depression: A meta-analysis adjusting for publication bias.' *Journal of Psychiatric Research*, 77, (2016): 42–51.
3. Gordon, B. R., McDowell, C. P., Hallgren, M. et al., 'Association of Efficacy of Resistance Exercise Training With Depressive Symptoms: Meta-analysis and Meta-regression Analysis of Randomized Clinical Trials.' JAMA *Psychiatry*, 75(6), (2018): 566–76.
4. Sibley, B. A. and Etnier, J., 'The Relationship between Physical Activity and Cognition in Children: A Meta-Analysis.' *Pediatric Exercise Science*, 15(3), (2003): 243–56.
5. Dik, M., Deeg, D. J. H., Visser, M. and Jonker, C., 'Early life physical activity and cognition at old age.' *Journal of Clinical and Experimental Neuropsychology*, 25(5), (2003): 643–53.
6. Pajonk, F.-G., Wobrock, T., Gruber, O., et al., 'Hippocampal plasticity in response to exercise in schizophrenia.' *Archives of General Psychiatry*, 67(2), (2010): 133–43.
7. Erickson, K. I., Voss, M. W., Prakash, R. S., et al., 'Exercise training increases size of hippocampus and improves memory.' *Proceedings of the National Academy of Sciences of the United States of America*, 108(7), (2011): 3017–22.
8. Déry, N., Pilgrim, M., Gibala, M., et al., 'Adult hippocampal neurogenesis reduces memory interference in humans: opposing effects of aerobic exercise and depression.' *Frontiers in Neuroscience*, 7, (2013): 66.
9. Xu, B., 'BDNF (I)rising from exercise.' *Cell Metabolism*, 18(5), (2013): 612–14.
10. Cheng, S.-L., Yang, F.-C., Chu, H.-T. et al., 'Incongruent Expression of Brain-Derived Neurotrophic Factor and Cortisol in Schizophrenia: Results from a Randomized Controlled Trial of Laughter Intervention.' *Psychiatry Investigation*, 17(12), (2020): 1191–99.
11. Schmitt, K., Holsboer-Trachsler, E. and Eckert, A., 'BDNF in sleep, insomnia, and sleep deprivation.' *Annals of Medicine*, 48(1-2), (2016): 42–51.
12. Seidler, K. and Barrow, M., 'Intermittent fasting and cognitive performance - Targeting BDNF as potential strategy to optimise brain health.' *Frontiers in Neuroendocrinology*, 65, (2022): 100971.
13. Blair, S. N. et al., Kohl 3rd, H. W., Paffenbarger Jr, R. S. et al., 'Physical fitness and all-cause mortality. A prospective study of healthy men and women.' *JAMA*, 262(17), (1989): 2395–401.
14. Lee, I.-M., Rexrode, K. M., Cook, N. R. et al., 'Physical Activity and Coronary Heart Disease in Women: Is "No Pain, No Gain" Passé?' *JAMA*, 285(11), (2001): 1447–54.
15. Lee, D. C., Pate, R. R., Lavie, C. J. et al., 'Leisure-Time Running Reduces All-Cause and Cardiovascular Mortality Risk' *Journal of the American College of Cardiology*, 64(5), (2014): 472–81.
16. Men's Health Forum, 'Walking: Science Confirms 10,000 Steps a Day', 13 September 2022, https://www.menshealthforum.org.uk/news/walking-science-confirms-10000-steps-day.

17. del Pozo Cruz, B., Ahmadi, M., Naismith, S. L. and Stamatakis, E., 'Association of Daily Step Count and Intensity With Incident Dementia in 78,430 Adults Living in the UK.' *JAMA Neurology*, 79(10), (2022): 1059–63.

18. Puterman, E., Weiss, J., Lin, J. et al., 'Aerobic exercise lengthens telomeres and reduces stress in family caregivers: A randomized controlled trial - Curt Richter Award Paper 2018.' Psycho-neuroendocrinology, 98, (2018): 245–52.

19. McPhee, J. S., French, D. P., Jackson, D. et al., 'Physical activity in older age: perspectives for healthy ageing and frailty.' *Biogerontology*, 17(3), (2016): 567–80.

20. Chilibeck, P. D., Sale, D. G. and Webber, C. E., 'Exercise and bone mineral density.' *Sports Medicine*, 19(2), (1995): 103–22.

21. Oudbier, S. J., Goh, J. et al., 'Pathophysiological Mechanisms Explaining the Association Between Low Skeletal Muscle Mass and Cognitive Function.' *The Journals of Gerontology: Series A: Biological Sciences & Medical Sciences*, 77(10), (2022): 1959–68.

22. Marques, A., Gomez-Baya, D., Peralta, M. et al., 'The Effect of Muscular Strength on Depression Symptoms in Adults: A Systematic Review and Meta-Analysis.' *International Journal of Environmental Research and Public Health*, 17(16), (2020): 5674.

23. Leal, L. G., Lopes, M. A. and Batista Jr., M. L., 'Physical Exercise-Induced Myokines and Muscle-Adipose Tissue Crosstalk: A Review of Current Knowledge and the Implications for Health and Metabolic Diseases.' *Frontiers in Physiology*, 9, (2018): 1307.

24. McTiernan, A., Friedenreich, C. M., Katzmarzyk, P. T. et al., 'Physical Activity in Cancer Prevention and Survival: A Systematic Review.' *Medicine & Science in Sports & Exercise*, 51(6), (2019): 1252–61.

25. Armour, M., Ee, C. C., Naidoo, D. et al., 'Exercise for dysmenorrhoea.' *Cochrane Database of Systemic Reviews*, 9(9), (2019): CD004142.

26. Baird, D. D., Dunson, D. B., Hill, M. C. et al., 'Association of physical activity with development of uterine leiomyoma.' *American Journal of Epidemiology*, 165(2), (2007): 157–63.

27. Vitonis, A. F., Hankinson, S. E., Hornstein, M. D. and Missmer, S. A., 'Adult physical activity and endometriosis risk.' *Epidemiology*, 21(1), (2010): 16–23.

28. Woodward, A., Klonizakis, M. and Broom, D., 'Exercise and Polycystic Ovary Syndrome.' *Advances in Experimental Medicine and Biology*, 1228, (2020): 123–36.

29. Tikac, G., Unal, A. and Altug, F., 'Regular exercise improves the levels of self-efficacy, self-esteem and body awareness of young adults.' *The Journal of Sports Medicine and Physical Fitness*, 62(1), (2022): 157–61.

30. 'UK Chief Medical Officers' Physical Activity Guidelines', 7 September 2019, https://assets.publishing.service.gov.uk/government/uploads/system/uploads/attachment_data/file/832868/uk-chief-medical-officers-physical-activity-guidelines.pdf

31. Palatini, P., 'Sympathetic overactivity in hypertension: a risk factor for cardiovascular disease.' *Current Hypertension Reports*, 3(suppl. 1), (2001): S3–9.

32. Masuo, K., Rakugi, H., Ogihara, T. et al., 'Cardiovascular and renal complications of type 2 diabetes in obesity: role of sympathetic nerve activity and insulin resistance.' *Current Diabetes Reviews*, 6(2), (2010): 58–67.

33. Perin, P. C., Maule, S. and Quadri, R., 'Sympathetic nervous system, diabetes, and hypertension.' *Clinical and Experimental Hypertension*, 23(1-2), (2001): 45–55.

34. Sata, Y., Head, G. A., Denton, K. et al., 'Role of the Sympathetic Nervous System and Its Modulation in Renal Hypertension.' *Frontiers in Medicine*, 5, (2018): 82.

35. Micieli, G., Tosi, P., Marcheselli, S. and Cavallini, A., 'Autonomic dysfunction in Parkinson's disease.' *Neurological Sciences*, 24 (suppl. 1), (2003): S32–4.

36. Alvares, G. A., Quintana, D. S., Hickie, I. B. and Guastella, A. J., 'Autonomic nervous system dysfunction in psychiatric disorders and the impact of psychotropic medications: a systematic review and meta-analysis.' *Journal of Psychiatry & Neuroscience*, 41(2), (2016): 89–104.

37. Kamphuis, M. H., Geerlings, M. I., Dekker, J. M. et al., 'Autonomic dysfunction: a link between depression and cardiovascular mortality? The FINE Study.' *European Journal of Cardiovascular Prevention and Rehabilitation*, 14(6), (2007): 796–802.

38. Maurer, J., Rebbapragada, V., Borson, S. et al., 'Anxiety and depression in COPD: current understanding, unanswered questions, and research needs.' *Chest*, 134(suppl. 4), (2008): 43S–56S.

39. Zaccaro, A., Piarulli, A., Laurino, M. et al., 'How Breath-Control Can Change Your Life: A Systematic Review on Psycho-Physiological Correlates of Slow Breathing.' *Frontiers in Human Neuroscience*, 12, (2018): 353.

40. Nair, S., 'Nasal Breathing Exercise and its Effect on Symptoms of Allergic Rhinitis.' *Indian Journal of Otolaryngology and Head and Neck Surgery*, 64(2), (2012): 172–6.

41. Petruson, B. and Theman, K., 'Reduced nocturnal asthma by improved nasal breathing.' *Acta Oto-Laryngologica*, 116(3), (1996): 490–2.

42. Cai, Y., Goldberg, A. N. and Chang, J. L., 'The Nose and Nasal Breathing in Sleep Apnea.' *Otolaryngologic Clinics of North America*, 53(3), (2020): 385–95.

43. Lin, L., Zhao, T., Qin, D. et al., 'The impact of mouth breathing on dentofacial development: A concise review.' *Frontiers in Public Health*, 10, (2022): 929165.

44. Lundberg, J. O., 'Nitric oxide and the paranasal sinuses.' *The Anatomical Record*, 291(11), (2008): 1479–84.

45. Martel, J., Ko, Y.-F., Young, J. D. and Ojcius, D. M., 'Could nasal nitric oxide help to mitigate the severity of COVID-19?' *Microbes and Infection*, 22(4-5), (2020): 168–71.

46. Ma, X., Yue, Z.-Q., Gong, Z.-Q. et al., 'The Effect of Diaphragmatic Breathing on Attention, Negative Affect and Stress in Healthy Adults.' *Frontiers in Psychology*, 8, (2017): 874.

47. Fernandes, M., Cukier, A. and Zanetti Feltrim, M. I., 'Efficacy of diaphragmatic breathing in patients with chronic obstructive pulmonary disease.' *Chronic Respiratory Disease*, 8(4), (2011): 237–44.

48. Jerath, R., Beveridge, C. and Barnes, V. A., 'Self-Regulation of Breathing as an Adjunctive Treatment of Insomnia.' *Frontiers in Psychiatry*, 9, (2019): 780.

49. Ferreira, J. B., Plentz, R. D. M., Stein, C. et al., 'Inspiratory muscle training reduces blood pressure and sympathetic activity in hypertensive patients: a randomized controlled trial.' *International Journal of Cardiology*, 166(1), (2013): 61–7.

50. Panja, A., *The Health Fix* (Short Books, 2023).

51. Sakuragi, S., Sugiyama, Y. and Takeuchi, K., 'Effects of laughing and weeping on mood and heart rate variability.' *Journal of Physiological Anthropology and Applied Human Science*, 21(3), (2002): 159–65.

52. Fujiwara, Y. and Okamura, H., 'Hearing laughter improves the recovery process of the autonomic nervous system after a stress-loading task: a randomized controlled' trial. *BioPsychoSocial Medicine*, 12, (2018): 22.

53. Weisenberg, M., Raz, T. and Hener, T., 'The influence of film-induced mood on pain perception.' *Pain*, 76(3), (1998): 365–75.

54. Shahidi, M., Mojtahed, A., Modabbernia, A. et al., 'Laughter yoga versus group exercise program in elderly depressed women: a randomized controlled trial.' *International Journal of Geriatric Psychiatry*, 26(3), (2011): 322–7.

55. Louie, D., Brook, K. and Frates, E., 'The Laughter Prescription: A Tool for Lifestyle Medicine.' *American Journal of Lifestyle Medicine*, 10(4), (2016): 262–7.

56. Dickerson, A. K., Mills, Z. G. and Hu, D. L., 'Wet mammals shake at tuned frequencies to dry.' *Journal of the Royal Society Interface*, 9(77), (2012): 3208–18.

57. Lynning, M., Svane, C., Westergaard, K. et al., 'Tension and trauma releasing exercises for people with multiple sclerosis – An exploratory pilot study.' *Journal of Traditional and Complementary Medicine*, 11(5), (2021): 383–9.

Sleep

1. Chattu, V. K., Manzar, M. D., Kumary, S. et al., 'The Global Problem of Insufficient Sleep and Its Serious Public Health Implications.' *Healthcare*, 7(1), (2018): 1.

2. Kline, C. E., Chasens, E. R., Bizhanova, Z. et al., 'The association between sleep health and weight change during a 12-month behavioral weight loss intervention.' *International Journal of Obesity*, 45(3), (2021): 639–49.

3. Wang, D., Li, W., Cui, X. et al., 'Sleep duration and risk of coronary heart disease: A systematic review and meta-analysis of prospective cohort studies.' *International Journal of Cardiology*, 219, (2016): 231–9.

4. Song, C., Zhang, R., Wang, C. et al., 'Sleep quality and risk of cancer: findings from the English longitudinal study of aging.' *Sleep*, 44(3), (2021): zsaa192.

5. Bubu, O. M., Brannick, M., Mortimer, J. et al., 'Sleep, Cognitive impairment, and Alzheimer's disease: A Systematic Review and Meta-Analysis.' *Sleep*, 40(1), (2017).

6. Cassoff, J., Wiebe, S. T. and Gruber, R., 'Sleep patterns and the risk for ADHD: a review.' *Nature and Science of Sleep*, 4, (2012): 73–80.

7. Zhai, L., Zhang, H. and Zhang, D., 'Sleep Duration and Depression among Adults: a Meta-Analysis of Prospective Studies.' *Depression and Anxiety*, 32(9), (2015): 664–70.

8. Rossman, J., 'Cognitive-Behavioral Therapy for Insomnia: An Effective and Underutilized Treatment for Insomnia.' *American Journal of Lifestyle Medicine*, 13(6), (2019): 544–47.

9. Medic, G., Wille, M. and Hemels, M. E. H., 'Short- and long-term health consequences of sleep disruption.' *Nature and Science of Sleep*, 9, (2017): 151–61.

10. Goldstein, A. N. and Walker, M. P., 'The role of sleep in emotional brain function.' *Annual Review of Clinical Psychology*, 10, (2014): 679–708.

11. Nagai, M., Hoshide, S. and Kario, K., 'Sleep Duration as a Risk Factor for Cardiovascular Disease – A Review of the Recent Literature.' *Current Cardiology Reviews*, 6(1), (2010): 54–61.

12. Ayas, N. T., White, D. P., Manson, J. E. et al., 'A Prospective Study of Sleep Duration and Coronary Heart Disease in Women.' *Archives of Internal Medicine*, 163(2), (2003): 205–9.

13. Okun, M. L., Coussons-Read, M. and Hall, M., 'Disturbed sleep is associated with increased C-reactive protein in young women.' *Brain, Behavior and Immunity*, 23(3), (2009): 351–4.

14. Spiegel, K., Leproult, R. and Van Cauter, E., 'Impact of sleep debt on metabolic and endocrine function.' *The Lancet*, 354(9188), (1999): 1435–39.

15. Cappuccio, F. P., Taggart, F. M., Kandala, N.-B. et al., 'Meta-analysis of Short Sleep Duration and Obesity in Children and Adults.' *Sleep*, 31(5), (2018): 619–26.

16. Gottlieb, D. J., Punjabi, N. M., Newman, A. B. et al., 'Association of Sleep Time with Diabetes Mellitus and Impaired Glucose Tolerance.' *Archives of Internal Medicine*, 165(8), (2005): 863–67.

17. Yaggi, H. K., Araujo, A. B. and McKinlay, J. B., 'Sleep Duration as a Risk Factor for the Development of Type 2 Diabetes.' *Diabetes Care*, 29(3), (2006): 657–61.

18. Besedovsky, L., Lange, T. and Haack, M., 'The Sleep-Immune Crosstalk in Health and Disease.' *Physiological Reviews*, 99(3), (2019): 1325–80.

19. Dimitrov, S., Lange, T., Gouttefangeas, C. et al., 'Gα_s-coupled receptor signaling and sleep regulate integrin activation of human antigen-specific T cells.' *Journal of Experimental Medicine*, 216(3), (2019): 517–26.

20. Howie, E. K., Joosten, J., Harris, C. J. and Straker, L. M., 'Associations between meeting sleep, physical activity or screen time behaviour guidelines and academic performance in Australian school children.' *BMC Public Health*, 20(1), (2020): 520.

21. Shen, C., Luo, Q., Chamberlain, S. R. et al., 'What Is the Link Between Attention-Deficit/Hyperactivity Disorder and Sleep Disturbance? A Multimodal Examination of Longitudinal Relationships and Brain Structure Using Large-Scale Population-Based Cohorts' *Biological Psychiatry*, 88(6), (2020): 459–69.

22. Eugene, A. R. and Masiak, J., 'The Neuroprotective Aspects of Sleep.' *MEDtube Science*, 3(1), (2015): 35–40.

23. Horne, J. A., 'Sleep loss and "divergent" thinking ability.' *Sleep*, 11(6), (1988): 528–36.

24. Williamson, A. M. and Feyer, A. M., 'Moderate sleep deprivation produces impairments in cognitive and motor performance equivalent to legally prescribed levels of alcohol intoxication.' *Occupational & Environmental Medicine*, 57(10), (2000): 649–55.

25. Worley, S. L., 'The Extraordinary Importance of Sleep: The Detrimental Effects of Inadequate Sleep on Health and Public Safety Drive an Explosion of Sleep Research.' *Pharmacy and Therapeutics*, 43(12), (2018): 758–63.

26. Rosseland, R., Pallesen, S., Nordhus, I. H. et al., 'Effects of Sleep Fragmentation and Induced Mood on Pain Tolerance and Pain Sensitivity in Young Healthy Adults.' *Frontiers in Psychology*, 9, (2018): 2089.

27. Lacovides, S., George, K., Kamerman, P. and Baker, F. C., 'Sleep Fragmentation Hypersensitizes Healthy Young Women to Deep and Superficial Experimental Pain.' *The Journal of Pain*, 18(7), (2017): 844–54.

28. Bohra, M. H., Kaushik, C., Temple, D. et al., 'Weighing the balance: how analgesics used in chronic pain influence sleep?' *British Journal of Pain*, 8(3), (2014): 107–18.

29. Ju, Y. S., Ooms, S. J., Sutphen, C. et al., 'Slow wave sleep disruption increases cerebrospinal fluid amyloid-β levels.' *Brain*, 140(8), (2017): 2104–11.

30. Spira, A. P., Chen-Edinboro, L. P., Wu, M. N. and Yaffe, K., 'Impact of Sleep on the Risk of Cognitive Decline and Dementia.' *Current Opinion in Psychiatry*, 27(6), (2014): 478–83.

31. Chaput, J. P., Dutil, C. and Sampasa-Kanyinga, H., 'Sleeping hours: what is the ideal number and how does age impact this?' *Nature and Science of Sleep*, 10, (2018): 421–30.

32. Depner, C. M., Melanson, E. L., Eckel, R. H. et al., 'Ad libitum Weekend Recovery Sleep Fails to Prevent Metabolic Dysregulation during a Repeating Pattern of Insufficient Sleep and Weekend Recovery Sleep.' *Current Biology*, 29(6), (2019): 957–67.

33. Willich, S. N., Löwel, H., Lewis, M. et al., 'Weekly variation of acute myocardial infarction. Increased Monday risk in the working population.' *Circulation*, 90(1), (1994): 87–93.

34. Aboyans, V., Cassat, C., Lacroix, P. et al., 'Is the morning peak of acute myocardial infarction's onset due to sleep-related breathing disorders? A prospective study.' *Cardiology*, 94(3), (2000): 188–92.

35. Fares, A., 'Winter Cardiovascular Diseases Phenomenon.' *North American Journal of Medicine and Science*, 5(4), (2013): 266–79.

36. Sandhu, A., Seth, M. and Gurm, H. S., 'Daylight savings time and myocardial infarction.' *Open Heart*, 1(1), (2014): e000019.

37. Laffan, J. et al. Data presented at the British Cardiovascular Society (BSC) conference. Reported by British Heart Foundation, 'Why are serious heart attacks more likely on a Monday?', 9 June 2023. https://www.bhf.org.uk/information-support/heart-matters-magazine/news/behind-the-headlines/heart-attack-monday

38. Underwood, E., 'Neuroscience. Sleep: the brain's housekeeper?' *Science*, 342(6156), (2013): 301. Erratum in *Science*, 343(6170), (2013): 486.

39. Reddy, O. C., van der Werf, Y. D., 'The Sleeping Brain: Harnessing the Power of the Glymphatic System through Lifestyle Choices.' *Brain Sciences*, 10(11), (2020): 868.

40. Xie, L., Kang, H., Xu, Q. et al., 'Sleep Drives Metabolite Clearance from the Adult Brain.' *Science*, 342(6156), (2013): 373–7.

41. Potter, G. D., Skene, D. J., Arendt, J. et al., 'Circadian Rhythm and Sleep Disruption: Causes, Metabolic Consequences, and Countermeasures.' *Endocrine Reviews*, 37(6), (2016): 584–608.

42. Schiavo-Cardozo, D., Lima, M. M. O., Pareja, J. C. and Geloneze, B., 'Appetite-regulating hormones from the upper gut: disrupted control of xenin and ghrelin in night workers.' *Clinical Endocrinology*, 79(6), (2013): 807–11.

43. Irwin, M., McClintick, J., Costlow, C. et al., 'Partial night sleep deprivation reduces natural killer and cellular immune responses in humans.' *The Federation of American Societies for Experimental Biology Journal*, 10(5), (1996): 643–53.

44. Lin, C.-L., Liu, T.-C., Wang, Y.-N. et al., 'The Association Between Sleep Disorders and the Risk of Colorectal Cancer in Patients: A Population-based Nested Case-Control Study.' *In Vivo*, 33(2), (2019): 573–79.

45. Cao, J., Eshak, E. S., Liu, K. et al., 'Sleep duration and risk of breast cancer: The JACC Study.' *Breast Cancer Research and Treatment*, 174(1), (2019): 219–25.

46. Sigurdardottir, L. G., Valdimarsdottir, U. A., Mucci, L. A. et al., 'Sleep Disruption Among Older Men and Risk of Prostate Cancer.' *Cancer Epidemiology Biomarkers & Prevention*, 22(5), (2013): 872–79.

47. Peever, J. and Fuller, P. M., 'Neuroscience: A Distributed Neural Network Controls REM Sleep.' *Current Biology*, 26(1), (2016): R34–5.

48. Feriante, J. and Araujo, J. F., *Physiology, REM Sleep* (StatPearls Publishing, 2023).

49. Patel, A. K., Reddy, V., Shumway, K. R. and Araujo, J. F., *Physiology, Sleep Stages* (StatPearls Publishing, 2022).

50. Burgess, H. J. and Eastman, C. I., 'Early versus late bedtimes phase shift the human dim light melatonin rhythm despite a fixed morning lights on time.' *Neuroscience Letters*, 356(2), (2004): 115–18.

51. Patke, A., Murphy, P. J., Onat, O. E. et al., 'Mutation of the Human Circadian Clock Gene CRY1 in Familial Delayed Sleep Phase Disorder.' *Cell*, 169(2), (2017): 203–15.

52. Stothard, E. R., McHill, A. W., Depner, C. M. et al., 'Circadian Entrainment to the Natural Light–Dark Cycle across Seasons and the Weekend.' *Current Biology*, 27(4), (2017): 508–13.

53. Cho, Y., Ryu, S.-H., Lee, B. R. et al., 'Effects of artificial light at night on human health: A literature review of observational and experimental studies applied to exposure assessment.' *Chronobiology International*, 32(9), (2015): 1294–310.

54. Farhud, D. and Aryan, Z., 'Circadian Rhythm, Lifestyle and Health: A Narrative Review.' *Iranian Journal of Public Health*, 47(8), (2018): 1068–76.

55. Voigt, R. M., Forsyth, C. B., Green, S. J. et al., 'Circadian Rhythm and the Gut Microbiome.' *International Review of Neurobiology*, 131, (2016): 193–205.

56. Chung, N., Bin, Y. S., Cistulli, P. A. and Chow, C. M., 'Does the Proximity of Meals to Bedtime Influence the Sleep of Young Adults? A Cross-Sectional Survey of University Students.' *International Journal of Environmental Research and Public Health*, 17(8), (2020): 2677.

57. Urry, E. and Landolt, H. P., 'Adenosine, caffeine, and performance: from cognitive neuroscience of sleep to sleep pharmacogenetics.' *Current Topics in Behavioral Neurosciences*, 25, (2015): 331–66.

58. Lovato, N. and Lack, L., 'The effects of napping on cognitive functioning.' *Progress in Brain Research*, 185, (2010): 155–66.

59. Souabni, M., Hammouda, O., Romdhani, M. et al., 'Benefits of Daytime Napping Opportunity on Physical and Cognitive Performances in Physically Active Participants: A Systematic Review.' *Sports Medicine*, 51(10), (2021): 2115–46.

60. Milner, C. E. and Cote, K. A., 'Benefits of napping in healthy adults: impact of nap length, time of day, age, and experience with napping.' *Journal of Sleep Research*, 18(2), (2009): 272–81.

61. Dautovich, N. D., McCrae, C. S. and Rowe, M., 'Subjective and Objective Napping and Sleep in Older Adults: Are Evening Naps "Bad" for Nighttime Sleep?' *Journal of the American Geriatrics Society*, 56(9), (2008): 1681–86.

62. Stutz, J., Eiholzer, R. and Spengler, C. M., 'Effects of Evening Exercise on Sleep in Healthy Participants: A Systematic Review and Meta-Analysis.' *Sports Medicine*, 49(4), (2019): 269–87.

63. Basso, J. C., McHale, A., Ende, V. et al., 'Brief, daily meditation enhances attention, memory, mood, and emotional regulation in non-experienced meditators.' *Behavioural Brain Research*, 356, (2019): 208–20.

64. Kim, D. Y., Hong, S.-H., Jang, S.-H. et al., 'Systematic Review for the Medical Applications of Meditation in Randomized Controlled Trials.' *International Journal of Environmental Research and Public Health*, 19(3), (2022): 1244.

65. Rusch, H. L., Rosario, M., Levison, L. M. et al., 'The effect of mindfulness meditation on sleep quality: a systematic review and meta-analysis of randomized controlled trials.' *Annals of the New York Academy of Sciences*, 1445(1), (2019): 5-16.

66. Shi, L., Zhang, D., Wang, L. et al., 'Meditation and blood pressure: a meta-analysis of randomized clinical trials.' *Journal of Hypertension*, 35(4), (2017): 696–706.

67. Lardone, A., Liparoti, M., Sorrentino, P. et al., 'Mindfulness Meditation Is Related to Long-Lasting Changes in Hippocampal Functional Topology during Resting State: A Magnetoencephalography Study.' *Neural Plasticity*, 2018, (2018): 5340717.

68. Black, D. S., O'Reilly, G. A., Olmstead, R. et al., 'Mindfulness meditation and improvement in sleep quality and daytime impairment among older adults with sleep disturbances: a randomized clinical trial.' *JAMA Internal Medicine*, 175(4), (2015): 494–501.

69. Nagendra, R. P., Maruthai, N. and Kutty, B. M., 'Meditation and Its Regulatory Role on Sleep.' *Frontiers in Neurology*, 3, (2012): 54.

70. Massion, A. O., Teas, J., Hebert J. R. et al., 'Meditation, melatonin and breast/prostate cancer: hypothesis and preliminary data.' *Medical Hypotheses*, 44(1), (1995): 39–46.

71. Bujatti, M. and Riederer, P., 'Serotonin, noradrenaline, dopamine metabolites in transcendental meditation-technique.' *Journal of Neural Transmission*, 39(3), (1976): 257–67.

72. Jahnke, R., Larkey, L., Rogers, C. et al., 'A Comprehensive Review of Health Benefits of Qigong and Tai Chi.' *American Journal of Health Promotion*, 24(6), (2010): e1–25.

73. Zeng, Y., Luo, T., Xie, H. et al., 'Health benefits of qigong or tai chi for cancer patients: a systematic review and meta-analyses.' *Complementary Therapies in Medicine*, 22(1), (2014): 173–86.

74. Kushlev, K., Hunter, J.,Proulx, J. D. E. et al., 'Smartphones reduce smiles between strangers.' *Computers in Human Behavior*,91, (2018): 12–16.

75. Karim, F., Oyewande, A. A., Abdalla, L. F. et al., 'Social Media Use and Its Connection to Mental Health: A Systematic Review.' *Cureus*, 12(6), (2020): e8627.

76. Muench, A., Vargas, I., Grandner, M. A. et al., 'We know CBT-I works, now what?' *Faculty Reviews*, 11, (2022): 4.

77. Raglan, G. B., Swanson, L. M. and Arnedt, J. T., 'Cognitive Behavioral Therapy for Insomnia in Patients with Medical and Psychiatric Comorbidities.' *Sleep Medicine Clinics*, 14(2), (2019): 167–75.

78. Doghramji, K., 'The epidemiology and diagnosis of insomnia.' *The American Journal of Managed Care*, 12(suppl. 8), (2006): S214–20.

Your *Get Well, Stay Well* Plan

1. Clear, J., *Atomic habits: An Easy & Proven Way to Build Good Habits & Break Bad Ones* (Random House Business, 2018).

2. Shnayder-Adams, M. M. and Sekhar, A., 'Micro-habits for life-long learning.' *Abdominal Radiology*, 46(12), (2021): 5509–12.

3. Fogg, B. J., *Tiny Habits: The Small Changes That Change Everything* (Virgin Books, 2020).

4. Hollingsworth, J. C. and Redden, D. T., 'Tiny Habits® for Gratitude – Implications for Healthcare Education Stakeholders.' *Frontiers in Public Health*, 10, (2022): 866992.

5. Rule of Three, 'What is the mysterious "rule of three"?', https://www.rule-of-three.co.uk/articles/what-is-the-rule-of-three-copywriting.

6. Monroy, M. and Keltner, D., 'Awe as a Pathway to Mental and Physical Health.' *Perspectives on Psychological Science*, 18(2), (2022): 309–20.

7. Keltner, D. and Haidt, J., 'Approaching awe, a moral, spiritual, and aesthetic emotion.' *Cognition and Emotion*, 17(2), (2003): 297–314.

8. Bell, J. T. and Spector, T. D., 'A twin approach to unraveling epigenetics.' *Trends in Genetics*, 27(3), (2011): 116–25.

9. Peng, H., Gao, W., Cao, W. et al., 'Combined healthy lifestyle score and risk of epigenetic aging: a discordant monozygotic twin study.' *Aging*, 13(10), (2021): 14039–52.

10. Ornish, D., Lin, J., Chan, J. M. et al., 'Effect of comprehensive lifestyle changes on telomerase activity and telomere length in men with biopsy-proven low-risk prostate cancer: 5-year follow-up of a descriptive pilot study.' *The Lancet Oncology*, 14(11), (2013): 1112–20.

11. Stenblom EL, Egecioglu E, Landin-Olsson M, Erlanson-Albertsson C. Consumption of thylakoid-rich spinach extract reduces hunger, increases satiety and reduces cravings for palatable food in overweight women. Appetite. 2015 Aug;91:209-19. doi: 10.1016/j.appet.2015.04.051. Epub 2015 Apr 17. PMID: 25895695.

Index

About the Author

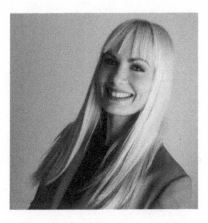

Photo credit: Ali Geromoschos

Dr Gemma Newman has been a British family doctor for twenty years. She is also a member of the British Society of Lifestyle Medicine, a founding member and ambassador for Plant Based Health Professionals UK and a Reiki healer. Her holistic health, nutrition and lifestyle advice has achieved tremendous results for her patients, as well as numerous others via her @PlantPowerDoctor Instagram platform.

She is regularly invited to teach other doctors and the general public about the benefits of plant-based nutrition via training programs, podcasts and medical conferences. Dr Newman has been featured on ITV, Channel 4, Channel 5 and Sky News Sunrise as well as BBC Radio. She has contributed to numerous articles for magazines, newspapers and podcasts. She has written two books: *The Plant Power Doctor* (Ebury, 2021) and *Get Well, Stay Well* (Ebury, 2023).

Connect with Gemma on Instagram and Facebook @plantpowerdoctor and via her website gemmanewman.com

Notes and Journalling Pages

Notes and Journalling Pages

Notes and Journalling Pages

Notes and Journalling Pages

Notes and Journalling Pages

Notes and Journalling Pages

Notes and Journalling Pages

Notes and Journalling Pages

Notes and Journalling Pages

Notes and Journalling Pages

Notes and Journalling Pages